SELF-HELP
OSTEOPATHY

SELF-HELP OSTEOPATHY

Robert Bowden BA, DO, MNZRO

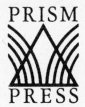

PRISM
PRESS

First published in Australasia in 1988 by
Nature & Health Books,
This edition co-published in Great Britain by
Prism Press, 2 South Street, Bridport,
Dorset DT6 3NQ, England
and distributed in the United States of America by
the Avery Publishing Group Inc.,
350 Thorens Avenue, Garden City Park, New York, 11040

ISBN 1 85327 014 8

Design: Craig Peterson
Artwork: Joanne Palme
Typeset by Deblaere Typesetting Pty. Ltd.
Printed in Australia by The Book Printer

CONTENTS

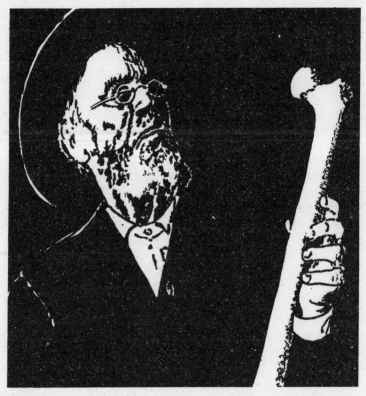

Doctor A. T. Still, the father of Osteopathy, in 1874

INTRODUCTION

Osteopathy is a system of manual medicine which complements the more ordinary healing professions and its professional health care gives an added dimension to personal well-being.

Registered osteopaths practise in their offices a science of osteopathic medicine using proven knowledge and methods accepted by allopathic medicine, combined with a distinctive philosophy which separates them from the strictly orthodox, that is, one based on the body's natural ability to balance itself. The professional doctor of osteopathy is skilled at correcting structural problems or osteopathic lesions such as poor posture, slight malpositions and limited movement of body parts. Such structural problems can affect nerves and blood-flow to various parts of the body including the internal organs.

At the beginning of the seventies, when I was a student at a college of osteopathic medicine, these therapies were called 'alternative', an unfortunate label that antagonised and threatened other medical doctors. With the demise of the Aquarian Age, osteopathy is now designated as 'complementary' to drugs and surgery. Today it is recognised as a valid system by the World Health Organisation which includes 'Osteopathic Lesion' as a listing in the International Classification of Disease.

Osteopathy dates back to 1874 in Missouri when orthodox medicine was much more primitive and backward than modern medicine is today. It was the eccentric discovery of an army surgeon, Andrew Taylor Still, M.D., and his basic concept still followed by osteopaths to this day was that 'structure governs function'. His unique idea that the framework of the body in its mechanical efficiency (or inefficiency) totally regulated the inner workings and harmony of all its organs and parts, was a radical breakthrough.

Many of the ideas in osteopathy are not only applicable professionally through manipulative therapy as developed by Dr Still, but also in the home as a form of self-help. Treatments such as exercise therapy and soft-tissue massage need not be performed solely by the osteopathic physicians, but can be practised safely by patients between regular treatments by their osteopathic doctor.

During the four years I was studying for my degree in osteopathy, it became apparent to me that the principles of this wonderful healing science have a vast potential for the health and happiness of everyone. Some aspects of osteopathy may be used as a base of self improvement and development towards health, and resistance to disease. This book has been designed to assist patients who will do well under osteopathic physicians, by offering ideas for ways to relieve these symptoms using non-invasive and drugless methods. Sufferers from asthma, migraine, R.S.I., low back or 'slipped disc' pain can assist themselves through osteopathic methods and much can be done to prevent osteopathic lesions occurring or progressing to be much more serious health problems.

Health is not just the absence of disease symptoms, but is a positive state of well-being on the physical, mental and spiritual levels of life. Osteopathy is a medical profession which serves humanity at a most profound level in society, and is a philosophy of healthy living which expresses the holistic awareness first announced by that American, Doctor Andrew Taylor Still in the Modern World.

1 LOW BACK PAIN

Low back pain is one of mankind's most common ailments. All of us tend to neglect our backs until one day, when we least expect it, our lower back 'goes out'. Although your osteopathic physician can guide you on the way to a healthy and pain-free body, you can improve your posture and learn ways to prevent back strain in your daily life. Importantly, only you can take responsibility – with advice from your osteopath – to follow a daily exercise programme to build strong supporting stomach and spinal muscles.

Ever since man had the nerve to assume the upright position, his lower back has suffered. In the human body the structural elements used by engineers for a suspension bridge (in the four-legged animals) have been converted by evolution into a skyscraper (in the bipedal Homo sapiens).

Humans do not have the structural advantage of walking on all fours like their ape-like ancestors, and therefore their lower backs must bear the brunt of the body's weight. The lower back has also inherited the ever-increasing stress of daily living in our civilisation, poor posture, lack of exercise and overeating. (I often tell my patients if they spent their days hanging out of trees eating bananas, their backs would be better off.) A healthy back is strong, flexible and pain-free. The chief function of your spine is to support your upper body, protect your spinal cord and allow flexibility and free movement.

The lower back or lumbar spine is composed of five vertebrae (L1 through to L5) with their associated discs, nerve roots, muscles and ligaments. The vertebrae and discs in your lower back have the greatest load to bear and are the largest. A healthy back is one properly aligned and supported by strong back, hip and abdominal muscles.

Pain begins when nerve endings receive abnormal stimulation. The brain, the complex computer which decodes all nerve impulses, interprets the stimulation as pain. In response to pain, back muscles often try to protect the back by going into spasm, forming a splint to keep the sore area immobile. This muscle spasm can cause pain if prolonged.

Since the bones, discs, ligaments and muscles of the back are supplied by many nerve endings, there are various conditions related to the osteopathic lesion which can cause back pain. In addition to the common physical causes, the stress, fatigue and anxiety of daily life can significantly increase low back pain.

The Causes of Back Pain

The osteopathic lesion is an area of poor or restricted mobility in the joints of the back, causing it to 'go out of place' and thus causing pain. Osteopathic lesions also cause other bodily complaints by interfering with the usual flow of nerve signals to and from the brain. Poor posture, lack of exercise and overeating can be your back's worst enemies and the cause of much ill health.

Most low back pain is a result of using the spine improperly. Poor posture strains the lower back and makes it more vulnerable. A swayback (lordosis, or increased lumbar curve) can result from weak muscles especially in the abdomen. Weak or flabby tummy muscles (pot bellies) deprive your back of its greatest support. Being overweight adds to the strain.

Back strain occurs when back muscles seize up. This usually occurs as a result of common activities done improperly such as bending, lifting, standing or sitting. The injury may also occur as a result of wrenching caused by an automobile accident or athletic injury. Back strain can heal completely if properly treated by an osteopathic physician, but practising proper back mechanics can prevent many back strains and would save millions of dollars in the workplace each year.

'Slipped' or 'ruptured' disc is a notorious diagnosis for a medical doctor to label severe pain and disability. The semi-solid centre of the intervertebral disc may 'slip', shift or bulge according to this theory, through its tough capsule, pressing on nerve endings. In extreme cases, the disc may rupture and herniate through the capsule (or annulus fibrosis), like a tire blow-out, and pinch the spinal nerves (a 'pinched nerve') or press on the spinal cord. If pressure or pinching of the spinal nerves continues, actual nerve damage can result with either numbness or muscle weakness in the legs.

Osteoarthritis is wear and tear in a joint due to a chronic osteopathic lesion. Osteoarthritis affects the discs and bones of the back in varying degrees with ageing. It narrows the discs and can cause irritating spurs on the vertebral bodies (osteophytes), which medical practitioners often point to on X-rays as a cause of pain. However, osteoarthritis is often present in your body with no discomfort at all. Proper use of your back and good posture can significantly decrease the wear-and-tear arthritis of ageing.

Tension and emotional problems of everyday living also play an important role in back pain. Economic worries, family pressure and fatigue can, in fact, cause muscle spasm. If you are willing to accept, understand and work to improve the emotional factors in your life, you will cope better with your back pain and improve your chances for a healthy back.

Miscellaneous causes in back pain include any condition of the body which affects spinal structures or nearby areas. Some, such as birth defects, and curvatures of the spine such as scoliosis, are uncommon. Others, like male prostate trouble or 'female problems' are not so rare. Spondylosis is a label for degenerative changes of the spine, and spondylolisthesis occurs sometimes in the lower lumbar spine and involves one vertebra shifting forward on another. Any severe or persistent backache should be brought to the attention of your registered osteopath or another qualified practitioner.

Posture and Exercise

It is important to learn and practise good posture and body mechanics. Maintaining a good lumbar curve is important to good back care. Test your posture by standing with your back against a wall – there should be only a minimal space between your back and the wall. A lazy, slouched posture or the 'military' position of a rigidly erect spine both increase the curves in your back.

Many people develop poor posture early in life. Teenagers may tend to slouch to be 'cool' and tall girls and boys may try to look shorter by slumping. Short people try to look tall and generally have good posture. Good posture *does* prevent backache.

• Straighten the curve in your neck by standing tall with your chin slightly tucked in. Tuck in your stomach and move your pelvis so that the curve of your back is partially reduced. Tighten the muscles in your buttocks and bend your knees slightly.

The following rest positions can relieve your back by moving the pelvis and straightening the spine:

• (At work or home) Stand in a comfortable position. Place your hands in the low back area and bend backwards. Hold for thirty seconds to one minute.

• (At work or home) Lean forward in your chair and lower your head to your knees for two to five minutes.

• (At home) Lie on your back, flat on the floor and place your legs on a low chair or stool. A pillow under your calves will make you more comfortable. For maximum relief, this position should be held for fifteen minutes.

Next to good posture and a willingness to help your back, the greatest support you can give your back is building strong and flexible supporting muscles, through a good exercise programme.

The role of your back muscles resembles that of guide wires supporting a tent. If the wires are strong and taut the tent will be stable – even in strong wind. If the wires are loose and frayed however, the tent will collapse or, in the case of your spine, sway-back may result.

Many people develop back curvatures through the lazy habit of resting their weight on one leg while standing for any length of time, or by tightening the muscle of the pelvis called the piriformis, by crossing one leg over another when watching television in a lounge chair. Even walking on the uneven canter of a city pavement (so designed to allow rainwater to drain) may cause imbalance of the pelvis and hips.

Before you start any therapeutic exercise programme, a complete evaluation by an osteopathic physician is recommended so that the correct exercises for your individual back problem can be selected, and osteopathic manipulative therapy used to fix the alignment of your spine as far as possible.

Prevention is Better than Cure

When lifting with your back, always bend your knees, not your spine. Lift with your legs and hold the object close to your body. Lift objects only chest high. When a load is heavy, get help and plan ahead to avoid sudden load shifts. Always be sure of your footing. Do not bend over with legs straight, or twist while lifting. Avoid trying to lift above shoulder level, as this position may cause injury.

While standing ironing or at the kitchen sink, do so with one foot up and don't slouch, with your body weight constantly on one leg. Always walk with good posture, keeping your head high, chin tucked in, pelvis forward, toes straight ahead. Wear sensible shoes and don't wear high-heeled or platform shoes when standing or walking for long periods.

Before driving, move the car seat forward to keep your knees bent and higher than your hips. As most car seats are very poorly designed, a small cushion or 'lumbar roll' behind the lumbar curve may be helpful. After a manipulative treatment by a registered osteopath, it is good to walk around the block for twenty minutes to allow the adjustment to settle in before sitting in the car seat to drive your vehicle. If you drive too soon after the manipulation it may negate the benefit of the osteopathic treatment.

Don't drive sitting far back from the wheel. Stretching for the pedals and wheel increases low-back curve and strain. At work, sit in chairs low enough to place both feet on the floor with knees higher than hips and sit firmly against the back of the chair. Do not slump or sit in a chair that is too high or too far from your work – avoid leaning forward or arching your back.

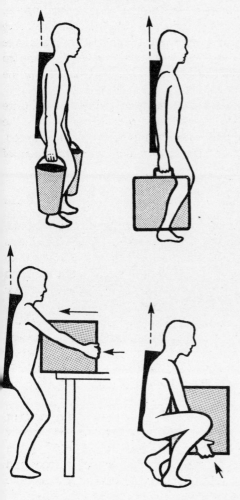

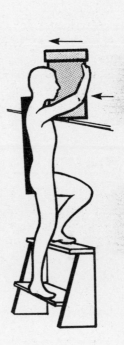

These are correct postures for lifting and carrying loads, avoiding back injury or the so-called 'slipped disc'

A good night's sleep on a firm mattress is good for you and your back. Sleep on your side with your knees bent and a pillow firm and fat enough to keep your head level with your shoulders to protect the alignment of your neck, or sleep on your back with a very thin pillow and another under your knees. Don't sleep on your stomach or lounge on soft, sagging, no-support mattresses or cushions for sway-back or back strain will result. Because we spend one-third of our lives lying down, it is important that we attempt to minimise stress while resting.

If we spend on average eight hours each night sleeping, then it follows that over a lifetime we spend as much as one-third of our time in bed. It is therefore essential that we lie on a bed which is not going to cause any harm to our body (and spine in particular) when resting. When choosing a bed we should look for:

- A bed and base sold together – not just a mattress only
- The base should be on rollers so that if you wish to shift the bed for some reason, it can be done relatively easily
- The base of the bed should be solid – it should not be a wire or sprung base; the mattress itself provides comfort
- The mattress should be firm enough to support your body when you lie on the edge of the mattress and firm enough to prevent you and your partner (if the bed is shared) from rolling together
- The mattress should have just enough 'give' so that when lying on your side, your hips and shoulders sink in slightly and your spine remains straight. Also, when lying on your back, your buttocks and shoulders should be cushioned, thus maintaining the normal curves in your spine
- The mattress should be ideally designed so that it need not be turned over to distribute wear
- The mattress should come with a guarantee to cover manufacturing defects. If possible, have the bed delivered and installed by the retailer
- Ideally try out the mattress – some stores may allow you to try out the bed of your choice for several days before buying. At the very least, lie on the mattress at the store.

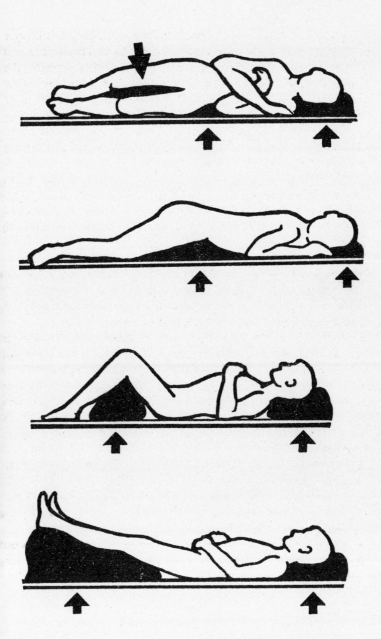

Comfortable resting positions when you have a bad back or 'slipped disc'

Many patients suffering from low back pain consult a chiropractor for spinal manipulation, and indeed, in remote areas not served by an osteopathic physician this may be very wise. Chiropractic therapy is most effective for recent strains of the back and neck, although it doesn't use any soft-tissue massage for muscles and ligaments. (Chiropractors are registered in the United States, Australia and New Zealand and you can be sure that a chiropractor has completed professional training in these countries. There is no legal register of chiropractors in the United Kingdom, however.)

It is a commonly held belief that spinal adjustment was discovered by a tradesman named David Daniel Palmer in Davenport, Iowa in 1895. Palmer claimed that he cured the deafness of a caretaker, Harvey Lillard, by restoring his hearing with a thrust to his back, releasing a trapped nerve pinched by subluxation.

Manipulation however, was announced by Dr Andrew Taylor Still in 1874 when he went on to found the American School of Osteopathy in Kirksville, Missouri. Kirksville records show that Mr D. D. Palmer came to Dr Still for treatment in 1893 and that he stayed there for six weeks. The following year he announced that he had independently discovered the method he called 'chiropractic' and started up the now famous Palmer College of Chiropractic.

Cynical osteopathic physicians often commented that chiropractic was the first six weeks of osteopathy. However, the osteopathic profession has never concentrated on the spine like many chiropractors, nor do they routinely X-ray every patient. Osteopathic physicians use X-rays less frequently, preferring to make their diagnosis by the skilled use of palpation with their hands to examine the back.

Osteopathic physicians also differ from physiotherapists in that they are trained to *diagnose* back problems. Physiotherapists do not do this and instead they carry out the instructions of a medical practitioner. Unlike doctors of osteopathy, physiotherapists also commonly use a whole range of machine equipment for their treatment.

2 MIGRAINES

Migraine headache is an exceptionally painful paroxysmal disorder that is very common among both adults and children. Onset occurs most commonly in the second and third decades of life, with frequent remission of the headaches after the age of fifty. It is more frequent in women than men and often there is a family history of migraines.

Ordinary headaches are quite different from migraine syndromes. Migraine symptoms are distinguished by the frequent association of periods of depression, irritability, disturbances of vision such as sensitivity to bright lights and difficulty focussing, nausea, vomiting and occasional numbness. Symptoms other than the headache are probably due to constriction of the blood vessels inside the head; and the headache itself (cephalalgia) to expansion of blood vessels of the scalp or the dura mater (one of three membranes supporting the brain).

Left untreated, a migraine attack may last for hours or even days; and the unfortunate sufferer often desires to be in a warm dark room and left alone. The headache often only affects one side of the skull (hemicranial) but it also may be generalised. When the headache is hemicranial, it will not necessarily be the same side with each attack.

In the absence of serious disease pathology or abnormally formed blood vessels, the causes of migraine can be categorised as due to dietary triggers, stress, P.M.T. or osteopathic lesions particularly of the cervical spine. Often a combination of factors will be present before an attack can begin.

Dietary triggers are significant as a cause. In England, medical researchers have isolated thiacin, a factor found in various food, as being a trigger for migraine attacks. Suspect foods include oranges, chocolate, cheese, coffee, pork and alcohol of any sort. However, not all of these foods will necessarily trigger an attack in an individual patient – a process of trial and error may be needed to identify the causative agent.

Stress, where commonly present, may bring on a migraine attack. The effects of excessive stress are virtually epidemic in our industrialised Western society and it will certainly make any form of headache worse. 'Weekend migraine' types generally result when a person under stress all week, paradoxically has the chance to unwind and relax for a while.

Premenstrual tension occurs most frequently in women between the ages of twenty-five and forty years and is often associated with headaches and migraine. Increased hormonal activity in the latter half of the menstrual cycle causes fluid retention in the tissues generally, and may affect the nervous tissue and the cerebral tissue. Cranial osteopathy or gentle manipulation of the sutures or joints of the skull may help in these cases. Cranial manipulation improves the flow of cerebrospinal fluid, relieving fluid pressure of the vault, and improves the function of the pituitary gland at the base of the brain. The pituitary gland rests in the floor of the skull and governs the endocrine system and hormone regulation (the endocrine glands release hormones that stimulate body functions and metabolism). Carried out by a trained cranial osteopath, manipulation of the skull is very gentle.

Osteopathic lesions are described as restrictions of movement in one or more of the joints of the body, most particularly the spine. This restriction results mostly in a very slight change of position or asymmetry of the vertebrae concerned, although the bones are still within their normal range of mobility. Changes of muscle tone also occur where paraspinal muscles go into spasm around the offending spinal segment.

Osteopathic treatment of migraine is based on a holistic philosophy and is best aimed at removing as far as possible the aetiological factors. Treating symptoms alone with drugs or whatever is at best palliative and does not prevent a recurrence of the condition. Dietary triggers must be avoided; where possible, stress must be reduced or relieved and osteopathic manipulative therapy (O.M.T.) utilised to correct impingements in the spinal column. A definite reduction in frequency and intensity of pain was found to result from the osteopathic normalisation of the neck when research into migraines was conducted at the British College of Naturopathy and Osteopathy in London in the early 1970s. When treating cases of headache (as opposed to migraine) which have been suffered for many years, the osteopathic physician often finds that the patient needs only one treatment session.

Of particular importance in the osteopathic treatment of migraine are the upper two vertebrae in the cervical column, called the axis and atlas. These two vertebrae when restricted in their movements, exert an effect on the part of the autonomic nervous system which controls the dilation and constriction of blood vessels of the scalp and interior of the skull (vasomotor nerves). Dilation and constriction of the pupils of the eye will also be affected.

The locking of the joint facets of the spine when an osteopathic lesion is present can be compared to the jamming of one drawer in a chest of drawers. A vertebra which normally moves freely becomes mechanically locked (or hypomobile) relative to other segments. The soft tissues and muscles tighten up to prevent further damage to the tender area of the back or neck and neurological effects result.

The vertebral artery is an important source of blood and oxygen to the brain and it runs through openings (or foramina) of the cervical vertebrae, across the atlas into the hole (or foramen magnum) of the skull. Asymmetry of the neck vertebrae may have a damming effect on blood circulation.

Lower down the spine, restrictions are generally found in the middle thoracic area (between the shoulder blades) and this is the area of the spine that provides the nerve supply (called the splanchnic plexus) to the stomach. Nausea and vomiting manifest when there are restrictions in this region.

As many patients present with a history of many years of migraine suffering before abandoning allopathic medicine in favour of a more natural approach, overnight results occur only occasionally. Immediate relief from pain is often afforded by osteopathic therapy, but a more lasting remission is generally only possible after a number of treatments. Neuromuscular therapy is essential in the relaxation of muscular tensions which perpetuate spinal lesions. The treatment of soft-tissue and muscle spasm using deep osteopathic massage is an effective preliminary to manipulation.

Many patients do not realise that the side-effects of overmedication with drugs used to combat migraine, are potentially as detrimental as the condition itself. Many of these drugs will produce side-effects of nausea, vomiting and headache when taken in excess.

Sometimes it becomes difficult to separate the symptoms from the side-effects. Properly conducted osteopathic treatment is completely natural and without the adverse effects potentially present with orthodox treatment. The osteopathic approach is treatment of the cause rather than the symptoms, and results are long lasting. The patient will often also benefit from an increased range of spinal movement, allowing a more energetic and fulfilling lifestyle.

The role of manipulative therapy in migraine has been controversial, but a review of differences of opinion depend upon whether the physician is disease-orientated or patient-orientated.

Self-Help for Migraine

The idea of self-help for migraine headaches is part of the foundations of the osteopathic profession initiated in 1874. In his autobiography, Andrew Taylor Still described one of the events which led him to the idea of manipulative therapy as the expression of the philosophy of osteopathy. Even as he used the drugs of his day, his mind had kept a record of his boyhood where he had suffered migraine: 'One day, when about ten years old, I suffered from a headache. I made a swing of my favourite plow-line between two trees; but my head hurt too much to make swinging comfortable, so I let the rope down to about eight or ten inches [21-25 cm] off the ground, threw the end of a blanket on it, and I lay down on the ground and used the rope for a swinging pillow. Thus I lay stretched on my back with my neck across the rope. Soon I became easy and went to sleep, and got up in a little while with the headache gone. As I knew nothing of the anatomy at this time, I took no thought of how a rope could stop a headache and the sick stomach which accompanied it. After the discovery, I roped my neck whenever I felt those spells coming on. I followed that treatment for twenty years before the wedge of reason reached my brain and I could see that I had suspended the action of the great occipital nerve, and given harmony to the flow of the arterial blood to and through the veins, and ease was the effect.'

Natural therapists often recommend herbal remedies such as chamomile, valerian or feverfew, for migraine. Valerian tea can be very effective but may also have side-effects of nausea or vomiting. Writing in a recent issue of the newsletter of the British Migraine Association, Dr William Thomson remarked that addicts of the herb feverfew would be interested to hear that 'their faith in this old herbal remedy is being confirmed'. A report in the *Lancet* from the research department of a drug company, had shown that feverfew has an action very like aspirin, in that it inhibits the production of prostaglandin in the body, 'the substance responsible for many of the aches and pains to which man (and woman) is heir'. This discovery, the drug company thought, would justify the plant's earlier reputation in herbals dating back to the time of the Anglo-Saxons.

One of the more interesting forms of prevention for migraine has recently been developed in New Zealand by Healthaire Research in Parnell, Auckland. In 1980 the use of 'negative ions' was reported in the results of double blind tests conducted in offices which showed that 'in a negatively-ionised office, the incidence of headaches fell from a quarter of those surveyed to about five per cent'. Healthaire generators can be easily used to negatively charge the home or office environment, enabling the body to assimilate oxygen more readily into the blood.

Sufferers with migraine tend to be hypoglycaemic (have low blood sugar) and do not metabolise sugar very well. When the sugar level in the blood becomes too low, the cranial blood vessels will expand and dilate to get more blood to the brain cells. This often leads to a headache, and therefore migraine victims should never miss a meal. Sufferers should eat at least three balanced meals a day, or even four or five smaller meals. The diet should emphasise complex carbohydrates such as whole grains, nuts and seeds, or whole potatoes (which release sugar slowly), and protein, while refined foods and simple carbohydrates such as white flour and sugar should be avoided. Fluid retention, particularly premenstrually, may provoke an attack, and women should watch their salt intake at this time.

A trigger point that has been used to relieve migraine is Colon 4, which is found in the fleshy mound of the hand between the thumb and first finger. Acupuncturists also claim that this point may relieve neck pain, headaches, toothaches, constipation, arthritis and neuralgia.

For patients with acute neck or arm pain, a neck collar may be very useful as a short-term help until your registered osteopath can be consulted. A collar can be medically prescribed but it is cheaper and easier to make one at home from tubular bandage and upholstery foam (see diagram on page 23). The use of a neck collar is inadvisable in the long-term however, as the continual immobilisation of any part of the body is contrary to the principles of osteopathy, and the collar should only be used as a temporary measure.

The use of local heat is very soothing and is applied to the neck or spine using a hot water bottle or heat pad. Alternatively, a cold pack may be tried as it can stimulate blood flow through a tight muscle in the neck. A small pack of frozen peas can be used to apply the therapy, but do not then eat the peas!

It has been discovered that the body produces its own drug store in the form of natural opiates called endorphins and encephalins, to control pain. Our mental attitudes have much to do with the brain's ability to control pain, and relaxation and stress reduction have much to do with the reduction of migraine. The discovery of these chemicals in the body is scientific confirmation of Andrew Taylor Still's basic idea that the human body is able to produce its own drugs and remedies when structurally and functionally sound. It was his idea that the patient is a natural laboratory who can be stimulated to produce his or her own cure.

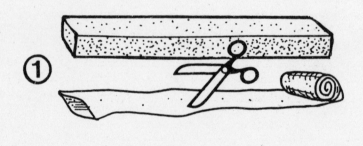

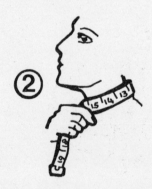

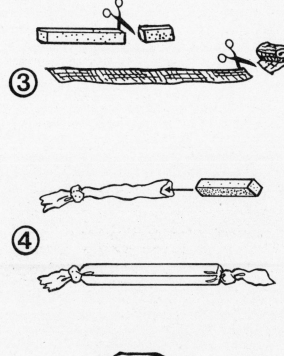

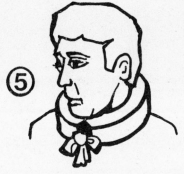

How to make your own cervical neck collar from tubular bandage and upholstery foam

3 ASTHMA, ITS SIGNS AND SYMPTOMS

A vague heavy tension in the chest and tightness with breathing is common in the early stages of asthma. There are several factors at work – some inborn, some emotional or psychological and some purely physical.

Many of the physical problems which underlie and predispose asthma, respond very well to qualified osteopathic manipulation of the spine, rib cage and skull. In remote areas, effective manipulation help from a registered osteopath may be difficult to obtain and parents may need to offer an asthmatic child some form of self-help.

In a severe asthmatic attack it is imperative to obtain professional assistance as 'status asthmaticus' is a dangerous and potentially fatal complication. However, between attacks, massage of the spinal and chest muscles is effective and safe in reducing occurrence of asthma. Gentle deep-tissue massage can be safely learnt and practised by non-professionals. Massage of the muscle masses along the thoracic vertebrae and the heads of the ribs where they attach to the spine, will lead to an awareness of the deep tension accumulated in the back and around the chest. Release of these soft-tissue spasms will assist breathing.

Overaction of the sympathetic nerves causes bronchial tube constriction and spasm as they stimulate the smooth muscles of the bronchioles. Breathing difficulties can be relieved by inhibiting the nervous irritation through firm massage. Inhibition is gained by deep steady pressure on the contracted fibres in the belly of a muscle, and this gives a positive feedback to the centres in the cord inside the spinal column. The masseur will also be able to feel for any obvious twist or deviation in the back with practice at massage, and any elevation of a rib head in particular, which should be looked at and treated by the patient's registered osteopath.

Asthmatic children often are consistent shallow breathers even when calm and apparently breathing normally. During quiet relax-ation sessions, deep respiration breathing with the diaphragm can be taught by the parent or therapist. Encouragement should be given constantly to breathe from the tummy rather than the upper lungs. The diaphragm is the large sheet of muscle which separates the chest and abdomen which contracts and relaxes as we take our breath normally. In asthmatics it is prone to spasm.

Subconsciously we build up layers of tight muscles in our back, chest and abdomen, the so-called 'body armour'. These are like the layers of an onion which can be 'peeled off' by soft-tissue massage.

This is why the neuromuscular or kinetic tissue manipulation used professionally by registered osteopaths is also effective in altering the noxious stresses in the structure of the body. Much of our body armour is psychological as we thoughtlessly tense ourselves when in emotionally threatening or stressful and unhappy parts of our lives. It is part of the primal 'fight or flight' reaction of mobilising the muscles for physical activity. When it is emotional stress there is often no outlet.

Soft-tissue massage is used more commonly by osteopathic physicians than other practitioners, before spinal adjustment. It consists of slow, deep controlled moves of the thumbs or the palmar surface of the fingers over connective tissues. It affects the ligaments, fascia and muscles, and the movements are, as far as possible, at right angles to the muscle fibres or the white fibres of ligaments and tendons. Its effects are said to be decongestion, restoration of muscle tone, increased range of motion of the joints and beneficial reflex effects on health problems.

In their search for the underlying cause of disease, osteopathic physicians make frequent recourse to the systems of reflex therapy such as acupuncture, zone therapy and Chapman's reflexes. Chapman's reflexes are palpable gangliform contractions or beads of lumpy feeling tissue which can be felt and located by the masseur through touch in specific body areas, and which can be related to disturbances of organs or glands. These contractions are particularly noticeable in the spaces between the ribs at the front of the chest, the abdominal muscles and beside the spine. Deep pressure will slowly remove them.

If a contraction has been present for some time however, it may have established an unhealthy reflex influence with a number of secondary trigger points in seemingly unrelated tissues. The findings of Dr Frank Chapman, D.O. are published in *An Endocrine Interpretation of Chapman's Reflexes* printed by the American Academy of Osteopathy. These are also known as neurolymphatic points in applied kinesiology, and those associated with the lungs are at the front of the body between the third, fourth and fifth ribs near the breastbone (sternum). Those in the back are between the third, fourth and fifth thoracic vertebrae, 25 mm to each side of the spine.

The diaphragm separates the body cavities and is responsible for healthy respiration. It attaches to ribs and the lower back, but surprisingly gets its nerve supply from the vertebrae of the neck. The phrenic

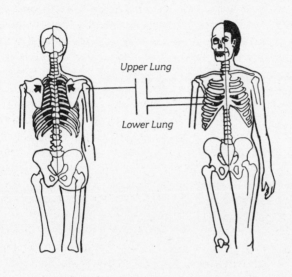

Upper Lung

Lower Lung

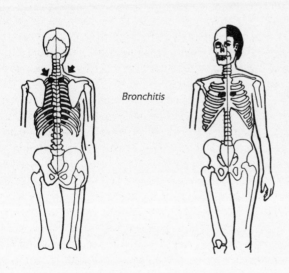

Bronchitis

Chapman's points for asthma relief

nerve passes through the cervical vertebrae and before birth, migrates into the chest cavity to supply the diaphragm. Massage of the neck is beneficial to relieve a contracted diaphragm.

Diagnosis by a registered osteopath will often find a spinal lesion of the fourth cervical in asthma cases. Specific adjustment of the neck should only be given by a registered osteopath, as neck manipulation by other practitioners has caused fatalities.

A holistic approach to the patient rather than an episodic one of treating the symptoms, is desirable for children with asthma. Skin tests and other procedures are often used to pinpoint the patient's allergic tendencies. Common offenders are pollen, animal hair, dust and foods. Proper nutrition is necessary and the asthmatic should eliminate from the diet those foods that may bring on an attack. A high fluid intake and the inhalation of steam may help to liquefy mucus and make it easier to expel it from the air passages. Osteopathic treatments such as thoracic pump, lymphatic drainage and diaphragmatic doming also assist in this.

Nutritionally, Vitamin A is necessary for the general health of the lungs and, together with Vitamin E, guards against visible and invisible air pollutants. The person should have a diet sufficient in the B-vitamin complex to avoid deficiency symptoms of nervousness, which might bring on an asthma attack. The need for Vitamin C is increased by stress and exposure to hot or cold weather, cigarette smoking and industrial air pollution.

Adrenal gland exhaustion is part of chronic asthma, and is worsened by steroid drug use. It can be partly countered with prescribed use of natural glandular extracts, Vitamin C and B5 (pantothenic acid).

The role of patient self-help and personal responsibility is vital for successful care of asthma – particularly for postural awareness, exercise and diet. However, with the links between asthma and spinal misalignments, registered osteopaths are opposed to the use of exercise as a form of treatment without professional guidance. Stretching and bending exercises may merely loosen already hypermobile joints, while areas of hypomobility (restriction) may become more fixed and jammed up. Once back alignment has been corrected by a registered osteopath, exercise systems such as yoga and tai chi are recommended as ways of maintaining mobility and tone. The role of the patient is not necessarily passive, and yoga exercises can be particularly helpful for asthmatics as they promote greater mobility of the spine and encourage deep breathing and relaxation.

Osteopathic physicians recommend any form of regular exercise which is enjoyable, uses a wide range of muscles and joints, and makes the lungs work to their fullest capacity. The British osteopathic profession has expressed concern about fitness and aerobics classes run by people with insufficient experience to discriminate between the various capacities of their pupils. Vigorous jerking motions can be hazardous to those who are susceptible to spinal lesions or back injuries. Patients, too, with a tendency to osteopathic lesions of the neck should not attempt neck and shoulder stands during the yoga class.

Psychologically, asthma is believed to be associated with the dominance of the lungs by the vagus or tenth cranial nerve. Repeated emotional conflict, striving and aggression, prepares the body physically to fight or run away due to the activity of the sympathetic nerves. On the other hand, the desire to withdraw from outwardly directed activity emphasises a parasympathetic tone which calls for a fulfilment of infantile dependent needs. Frustration of these needs causes onset of psychosomatic asthma, as emotions which are repressed and cannot be discharged through normal channels are converted to the asthmatic symptoms which serve partially as a release and partially as a defence against their expression. Many of these conflicts are laid down as the 'body armour' which tightens up our musculoskeletal tissues.

Exercises for Asthma

The first priority for the asthmatic patient is to breathe correctly. The patient should sit on a low chair, relaxing his shoulders and chest downwards, breathing in and out gently. The patient's tummy should swell as he breathes in and flatten as he breathes out. Feel for this tummy movement with your hand. Do not hold your breath or attempt any big breath in or out. Rest a little after each breath out. The patient should breathe like this most of the time.

Special positions for practising breathing

After exercise or when breathless, practise your breathing in these special positions: Standing with your elbows on a low table with your head on your hands; or crouching on the floor with your elbows on two stacked pillows and your head on your hands. Make it easy. Breathe a tiny bit faster through your mouth until you feel comfortable. If you breathe too much with your upper chest you will become hunched. The upper ribs will crowd together, forming a pigeon chest and the thoracic spine will develop a hump (kyphosis).

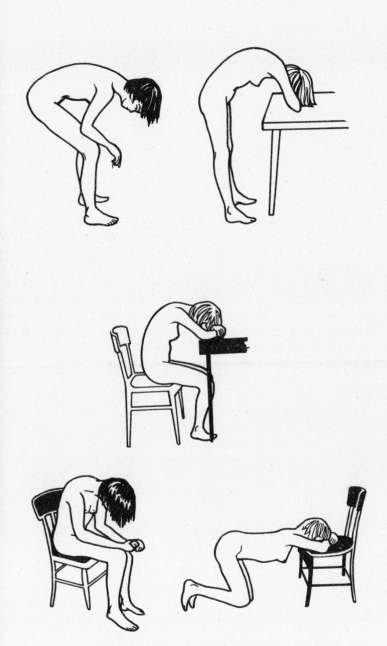

Resting postures during an asthma attack

Exercises to help your asthma

Every day, when you are not breathless, practise a few huffing exercises. Blow hard through a short tube. That sharp, wheezy noise is a 'huff'. You will soon learn to huff correctly without the tube.

● Lie on your side on a firm surface with two pillows under your lower back (i.e. downhill). Huff out your breath six times. Rest after every huff and practise gentle tummy breathing. Repeat on your other side.

Huffing is more effective as a way of loosening sticky mucus than coughing – but the huff should be short of a cough.

Gradually add other huffing exercises.

● Flap your arms ('wings') against your sides as you huff. Do this about six times. Small children can pretend they are geese, with lots of flaps and hissing!

● Bend over. Swing your arms from side to side. Occasionally huff, perhaps on every eighth swing. Swinging and swimming movements prevent your chest cage from stiffening.

● Sit cross-legged on the floor and put your fingers on your shoulders. Circle your elbows round and round like back-stroke swimming. This also helps keep you straight.

Status asthmaticus is an asthmatic crisis of sudden intense shock with breathlessness to the point of exhaustion and collapse. Professional assistance must be sought, and in these life-threatening situations drug therapy is justified. The resting position for status asthmaticus is high side lying on a mound of pillows with one pillow between the underneath arm and the body. Both knees should be drawn up.

Manipulative therapy by a registered osteopath may assist, but it should not be the high-velocity thrusting type adjustment. Functional techniques are an excellent therapy for the debilitated and exhausted patient. In some countries, osteopathic physicians have the right to use drugs as do the ordinary medical practitioners. However, asthmatics should not allow themselves to develop medication dependence due to the long-term overuse of cortisone. When the patient is coming off steroids, these should be withdrawn *very slowly* and under professional supervision.

Many asthma deaths in Australia and New Zealand are due to the excessively rapid withdrawal from steroids, with adrenal gland collapse after hospitalisation. Cranial osteopathy has much to offer

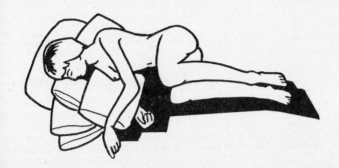

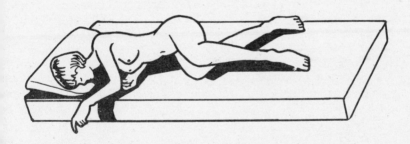

Try these resting positions during a severe asthma attack or 'status asthmaticus'

the chronic cases. To show how the mechanical and structural factors can dramatically influence the asthmatic condition, a case history in *General Practitioner*, July 1983, entitled 'Osteopathy cures Chronic Asthma' is very interesting.

It described the case of James Tweedie, aged eight, whose mother, a West London general practitioner, had tried conventional methods as well as hypnotism and acupuncture to help her son. He had developed asthma when he was four and none of the treatments had helped.

James was both asthmatic and bronchitic and his mother ascribed his condition to a mixture of allergic and emotional factors. He was degenerating when she decided to send him for osteopathic treatment at the British School of Osteopathy, near Trafalgar Square, in London.

He had weekly sessions and was treated on the spine, rib cage, shoulders, neck and skull. Within five months the asthma was cured – and as a bonus, his height increased dramatically. His schoolwork improved and, says his mother, he became 'a much nicer person to live with'.

Whatever allergic and emotional factors were involved, neither were able to operate without the structural component. After osteopathy, the child's body was able to function properly in response to stress. It no longer reacted to emotional stimuli or allergies with an asthma attack.

The osteopathic mechanism in asthma is twofold: Firstly osteopathic manipulative therapy helps the rib cage to move freely in respiration (no machine can function properly unless it is in a structurally normal state). Most asthmatics have poor posture and crowded rib cages and therefore they are unable to breathe normally, even when they are not in the middle of an attack. Correcting rib function is often easier with a child than an adult. The cranial osteopathic manipulation of the suture joints of the head also assists respiration by using what is known as the primary respiratory mechanism between the skull and the sacrum, the triangular bone at the base of the back. The sutures are the joints of the flat bones of the vault of the skull and they move slightly to allow the circulation of fluid bathing the brain and spinal cord (cerebrospinal fluid). The founder of cranial osteopathy, Dr William Gerner Sutherland, D.O., gave this regular movement of the skull the title 'primary respiratory mechanism' because it seemed the body's pendulum used to regulate other cycles and respiratory motions. Cranial osteopathy balances body functions throughout the system of the patient.

Secondly, osteopathy works through the normalisation of the spinal areas from which nervous control of breathing mechanism emanates. If a segment of nerve endings inside the spinal cord becomes irritable because of injury or poor posture, then any stimulus or stress to the body will affect that particular area more powerfully than the others. This is known as nerve facilitation and it is a major reason for the maintenance of many chronic conditions. The term 'facilitation' was coined by Professor Irwin Korr, Ph.D., who has conducted thirty-eight years of basic research, mostly at the Kirksville College of Osteopathy and Surgery in the United States.

By normalising the spinal mechanics and correcting osteopathic lesions in the back, osteopathic treatment reduces bombardment of nerve signals to the nerves controlling the breathing apparatus. From the orthodox medical viewpoint, the underlying disease pathology in asthma is believed to be nervous, through an imbalance between the sympathetic and the parasympathetic nervous systems. Osteopathic research confirms this belief in the knowledge that emotional, mental, allergic, irritative, postural and other factors can affect visceral organs such as the lungs, through lesioned spinal segments.

In asthma, autonomic imbalance is due to lesion of the vagus nerve, which produces bronchial-constriction and oversecretion of mucus; while osteopathic lesions in the spine or ribs affect vasomotor nerves to the lungs (which control blood circulation), causing a state of mucosal swelling, fluid retention and lowered function. When you are not breathing properly because your ribs are not functioning properly, your lungs become congested. So one of the most important osteopathic techniques is to adjust specific ribs.

Research carried out in London by Richard Carruthers, D.O., with asthmatics who have been treated either by osteopathy alone, or in combination with a natural diet, has shown that in the first approach there was a 70 per cent improvement rate, and in the latter approach (together with nutritional advice) there was a 61 per cent improvement rate. Cases under study included patients with extremely serious conditions who had required hospitalisation.

Any person seriously interested in the use of osteopathy as a treatment for disease would do well to study the written works of Dr Andrew Taylor Still. It was Dr Still who placed the science of manipulative medicine for conditions such as asthma on a scientific basis, and his founding of osteopathy came twenty years before any parallel system such as chiropractic.

When writing about asthma in his volume *Research and Practice* 1919, Dr Still said: 'As a mechanic I examined the union of ribs with the spine and in many cases, particularly on the right side at about the fifth, sixth, seventh and eighth, some or all of these ribs were off-centre . . . Also the muscles were in an abnormal condition in this and other parts of the spine, lower down and higher up.'

Dr Still then described a technique for the adjustment of the ribs with the spine and their articulations, with the breastbone at the front (unlike chiropractic, osteopathic manipulation is not just adjustment of the spinal bones) and the loosening of all the muscles and ligaments of the ribs. Dr Still then goes on with this advice: 'I want to emphasise to you each and all, that if you pull and haul your asthmatic patient every day, you will surely fail. For a day or two after treatment some of my patients report that they have coughed up as much as one pint [500 ml] of ropy substance in twelve hours. This is evidence that the lung is again beginning to do good work . . . During the past thirty years I have treated many asthmatics and have had no failures except one or two which were far gone with tuberculosis. In regard to diet I have no advice to give, further than to allow such patients to eat what they want of good plain nutritious food.'

4 R.S.I. – 'THE TERMINAL DISEASE'

Repetitive strain injury (R.S.I), the white-collar crippler, is a burgeoning plague among keyboard operators in particular. Many labels are applied to R.S.I., depending on the origin of the causal influence in vocational and leisure pursuits involving repeated motion, continuous vibration or protracted periods of positional tension.

Anyone with a tendency to the occurrence of osteopathic lesions at the junction of their rib-cage and neck, who uses their muscles excessively by doing a lot of repeated movement (as in fast and constant typing at a visual display unit), is prone to R.S.I. A common repetitive strain injury is tenosynovitis, a painful inflammation of the sheath connecting the tendons in the arm, wrist and fingers. For computer operators, typists and data processors, R.S.I. is an awful nightmare commonly worsened by conventional medical mismanagement.

In Australia, tenosynovitis and carpal tunnel pain in the wrists is reaching epidemic proportions with one-sixth of the workforce using keyboards being affected. An American osteopathic physician, Dr Gordon Zing, wrote of the 'lymphatic model' for inflammation and disability of the limbs.

Lymph circulation is the waste disposal unit for the waste products which leak from muscles and tendons into the fluid between cell fibres during constant and repeated muscle work and contraction. These toxins (catabolites) must be drained from around body tissues by the lymph vessels and veins. Lymph vessels do not have valves like the veins and rely on postural integrity and exercise to prevent stagnation and to drain fluid back into the circulation. Congestive pooling of lymph in the lining of the muscles (fascia), tendons and ligaments, can predispose towards swelling and painful disability.

According to Australian medical researchers there are three types of repetitive strain injury. Type one involves swelling due to fluid accumulating in a tendon sheath and, as inflammatory fluid gives way to fibrin or scarring fibres, the distressing clicking (crepitus) happens in the wrist tendons. Common labels for the pain include carpal tunnel, ganglion, tennis elbow, rotator cuff and pinched nerve.

Even medical doctors have noted that neck pain is involved and it is often worse at night (due to the pressure of the pillow at the base of the spine, at the neck and the first rib). There is numbness of all the fingers and sensations of numbness and swelling in both arms. The medical profession recognises specific 'tender points' in the upper body with this type of R.S.I. Only the osteopathic profession has pioneered the use of neuromuscular technique to treat these trigger points.

Type two, mostly long-term rheumatic pain patterns is another common R.S.I. In addition to pain there can be numbness, poor grip-strength and diffuse aching of the limb. Medicos differentiate this type because the pain involves the hand and neck and is worse when the arm is used, with the symptoms usually not occurring at night. Doctors note these patients are tender in the mid-trapezius muscle, the base of the neck, the junction of the upper ribs to the breast-bone cartilage, the side of the elbow and the inside of the shoulder blade (scapula). Other symptoms include gastric intolerance to drugs, dizziness, nervousness, anxiety, irritable bowel or bladder, and tension headaches. All of these painful symptoms point to the underlying cause of the osteopathic lesion.

In studies using the electron microscope, gross disruption of fibres has been shown in the muscles in tender points. Doctors admit the importance of the role of the nervous system and their research is focussing on the nerve causes of R.S.I.

Type three is the basket classification into which they toss the unexplained cases involving inflammatory or degenerative soft-tissue lesions where the pain focus is worsened by psychological problems.

R.S.I. is not necessarily a new disease – the Roman doctor Galen reported wrist pain in a charioteer in A.D. 200. Galen cured the case with a neck adjustment, thinking that the pain in the wrist was due to a trapped nerve. Medical practitioners note the 'tender points' with R.S.I.

When Dr Frank Chapman entered the American School of Osteopathy, founded in 1892 by Dr Andrew Taylor Still, the prevailing thought in the school in that year, 1897, was that there was no sickness without a bony lesion. Dr Frank Chapman believed, after thirty years as a practising doctor of osteopathy (D.O.), that the lymphatic system had a profound influence on body functions; that blocking – partial or complete – of the lymph fluid stream by common colds and other infections, was responsible for the many phases of disease. Lymphatic vessels have no central pump like the heart for arterial blood, to propel fluid flow.

The Chapman's reflexes associated with circulation of the arms are found at the attachment of the pectoralis minor muscle to the third, fourth and fifth ribs at the front of the chest. At the back of the body, sore tight points will be found at the upper angle of the shoulder blade (scapula) beside the first, second and third ribs.

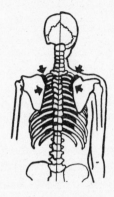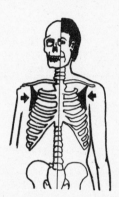

*Circulation
of arms*

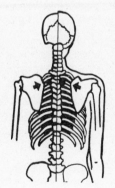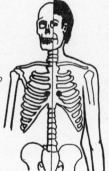

*Neuritis of
the upper limb*

These points are beneficial for RSI

Dr Chapman claimed that a point between the third and fourth ribs near the breast bone (sternum) will be found in association with extreme and excruciating pains in the nerves through the shoulder, arm, forearm, hands and fingers (as with type one, according to Chapman, 'more especially at night will the suffering be manifest'). At the back of the body a point for massage will be found 25 mm from the spine between the third and fourth thoracic vertebrae.

Chapman's interest in the lymphatic system was followed up by the research of Dr Gordon Zinc, D.O. (although now deceased, Dr Zinc was well known as a lymphomaniac!) and Dr Bernard Te Poorten, D.O. This investigation of the lymphatic circulation was conducted at the College of Osteopathic Medicine and Surgery in Des Moines, Iowa, at the University of Osteopathic Medicine and Health Sciences. Research indicates that congestive pooling (stasis) of lymph fluid causes the inflammation in diseases like R.S.I. Sufferers can be found to have an elevated first rib on the same side of the base of their neck as they first develop wrist pain. Osteopathic manipulation at the connection of the neck to the rib-cage and to the wrist is 80 per cent effective.

In the two-legged posture of man, the planetary rotation and gravitational strain of the Earth makes the spine prone to a twisting distortion, especially at the junction of the main back areas – the lumbar (loins), the thoracic (chest) and the cervical (neck). According to Zinc and Te Poorten, the common compensatory pattern (*fn) makes the first rib at the base of the neck commonly vulnerable to osteopathic lesion and misalignment. A strained first rib will block lymphatic flow. Occupational strains at poorly designed desks that are ergonomical disasters, and bad posture habits such as holding telephones between the head and shoulder while typing, are also responsible for blockage of normal lymphatic channels.

* The common compensatory pattern is an adaptation to the corkscrew effect of the Earth's gravity which contorts the spine into a spiral curvature (roto-scoliosis) in over 90 per cent of patients with back and arm pain. Registered osteopaths note the effects of the common compensatory pattern in the pelvis, at the first and fifth lumbar vertebrae, in the rib cage and at the junction of the atlas (first cervical vertebra) with the skull.

Exercise Plan to Reduce R.S.I.

Pelvic tilts – to help relieve lower back tightness and strengthen stomach muscles

Procedure: Sit at your terminal with your thighs parallel to the floor. Place one hand on your lower back and the other one low down in front of your abdomen, just above the pubic bones.

Action: Breathe in. As you breathe out, roll your lower back down so the pelvis tilts to lift the pubic bone up to the ceiling. Breathe well and pull in the abdominal muscles as you hold the position for a few seconds. Feel the curve of the lower back flatten out and the stomach muscles tighten. Return to start position and repeat as often as you like throughout the work day.

Shoulder lifts and rolls – to help relieve shoulder tightness

Procedure: Sit as before with your arms hanging loosely down by your sides.

Action: Breathe in and lift both shoulders up to the ears. As you breathe out, pull them strongly down. Repeat several times. Breathe well as you roll both shoulders forward and back several times. Feel the squeeze between the shoulder blades as you roll them back.

Back stretch – to stretch lower back muscles

Procedure: Start as above

Action: Breathe in as you lengthen your spine and as you breathe out tilt your pelvis, bend one leg and hold it under your thigh with your clasped hands as you hug it to your chest, trying to touch your forehead to your knee. Breathe well as you hold for a few seconds. Return to the start position and repeat the movement with the other leg. Repeat once more on each side.

Chest stretch – to help counteract rounded shoulders and encourage good posture and breathing

Procedure: As before with your back long, clasping your hands behind you just above your bottom. Palms face the ceiling and elbows remain bent.

Action: Breathe in. As you breathe out, squeeze your shoulder blades together so your elbows close towards each other. Feel the stretch across the chest and the contraction in the upper back. Repeat several times. Keep your shoulders down and level with your hands resting on your body. Make sure your lower back does not overarch.

Action: Breathe in as you lengthen your spine and as you breathe out turn your upper torso and head slowly and gently to one side, and as far as possible. Breathe well as you hold for a few seconds. Release and repeat to the other side. Keep the shoulders down and level as you twist your upper torso, and keep your hips and legs facing the front.

Neck releasers – to help release neck tension

Procedure: Always make sure your shoulders and upper back are warm before working on this area. Start as before.

Action: Turn your head *slowly* to look over your left shoulder. Return to the centre and repeat to look over your right shoulder. Return to the centre and lift your head to look at the ceiling – do not lower it back all the way. Return slowly to the centre and lower your head forward to take your chin towards your chest. Return to the centre and tilt your head slowly over to your right shoulder, until you feel a comfortable stretch on the left side. Return to the centre and repeat to the left side. Return to the centre. Keep your chin pulled in slightly to maintain length in your neck throughout the movement. Take it slowly and with control. Breathe well throughout.

Back stretch – to stretch upper back muscles

Procedure: Start as before but with your hands loosely clasped in front of your chest. Elbows are bent with the palms facing in.

Action: Breathe in as you lengthen your spine, and as you breathe out tilt your pelvis and at the same time invert your palms to stretch both arms out in front of your chest. Let your head drop forward as you do this. Breathe well as you hold this position before returning to start position. Repeat once more. Feel the stretch across the upper back, shoulders, and arms. Keep your shoulders down.

Body stretch – to stretch upper body and arms

Procedure: Start as before with your hands loosely clasped in front of your chest. Elbows bent with palms facing in.

Action: Breathe in as you lengthen your spine, and as you breathe out invert your palms and stretch both arms up to the ceiling. Breathe well as you hold this centred position, then emphasise the stretch a little to the right and then a little to the left. Return to centre and release your arms slowly down. Feel the stretch along the side of the body, particularly as you emphasise either side and along the arms.

Keep the shoulders down and pull in the abdominal muscles to prevent the lower back from overarching. Try not to twist as you stretch to the right and the left.

Spinal twist – to mobilise your spine
Procedure: Start as before with your back long, your feet hip-width apart and flat on the floor. Place your hands lightly on your chest with your elbows close to your waist.

SLIPPED DISCS

or many years before osteopathy was recognised legally and pro-
ssionally, the most common diagnosis with which patients turned
p at the surgery door of an osteopath physician was that of a 'slipped
sc'. Often these patients were in extreme pain and unable to walk,
nd it was the remarkable success of the osteopathic physicians
 these cases which was the basis of osteopathy's reputation with
ne public. Sadly, very few medical doctors have studied the bio-
nechanics of the human spine to the extent required to earn a degree
 osteopathic medicine. To the overworked and busy general prac-
tioner, more interested in germs and viruses, coughs and sniffles,
olds and flu, the general diagnosis for severe lower lumbar pain is
nat of a 'slipped disc'. However, it is quite impossible for a disc to
ctually 'slip'; there can be a rupture or a herniation which are
nislabelled as 'slipped'.

The disc that is supposed to slip is a tough cartilaginous ring that is
rmly attached to the spinal bones above and below and which looks
ke a doughnut with a dollop of cream in the centre. It contains an
nner pulpy mass, the 'nucleus pulposus'. If through wear or injury a
ear appears in the cartilage ring, the inner material can protrude.
his will cause cramp and spasm in the surrounding muscles and
vith pressure on the local nerves there will be very acute pain. The
nfortunate sufferer has great difficulty in standing erect and has
gonising pain shooting down one or both legs. This patient may
ave a true prolapsed intervertebral disc, or what is more likely, a
umber of other conditions such as a sacroiliac joint strain.

For the unlucky and gullible patient suffering from a strained
acroiliac joint in the lower back who is pronounced by the medical
pecialist or general practitioner to be suffering from a 'slipped disc',
fe becomes very unpleasant. After being dispatched to spend six
veeks in bed, the patient is squeezed into a cumbersome corset with
 constant diet of analgesics and anti-inflammatory drugs. He may
nd himself in a plaster cast or, in some cases, a risky surgical oper-
tion may be advocated. If the patient is suffering a prolapsed disc,
ne period in bed or wearing a corset will rest the lower back
ufficiently for some repair to occur. If the trouble is a strain or
steopathic lesion in the sacroiliac joint, however, these treatments
re worse than useless as the enforced immobility jams up the facets
f the back even further.

How is the osteopathic physician able to know, where other well-
neaning practitioners have failed?

A detailed history of the onset of the pain combined with past medical history, a careful palpatory examination (where the doctor of osteopathy uses the gentle tactile skills in his fingers to test tissue tone and mobility), a physical examination and possibly X-rays (where strictly necessary), will enable a registered osteopath to confirm or rule out the diagnosis of a 'slipped disc' with a great degree of certainty.

Once a disc is herniated there is no way of 'putting it back'. Any unqualified manipulation operator who claims to be able to replace a 'slipped disc' is, without doubt, not being completely truthful. With osteopathic manipulative therapy (O.M.T.) delivered by a registered osteopath it is possible to ease the pressure on the disc, then with gentle exercise and care, the slow repair can take place. In rare cases, surgery may be needed to remove the extruded pulp, but I would suggest surgery should be resorted to only after a registered osteopath has been consulted. Heavy-handed or quack adjustments can make a prolapsed disc much worse as the forceful type of manipulation can expel more of the disc nucleus. It is more important that you ensure that your osteopathic practitioner is fully registered for your own protection.

The effect of long-term unnatural wear and tear on the disc is to reduce the elasticity of the disc as a whole and to produce degeneration seen on an X-ray as narrowing of the disc space. The ability of the disc to act as a shock absorber is reduced, as well as loss of mobility and possibly pain and stiffness. It is therefore apparent that anything that can be done to prevent this all-too-common breakdown is desirable. Sensible exercise should be practised and a sensible diet followed, for being overweight is an added load to the spinal discs. Running or jogging on hard asphalt or concrete footpaths delivers violent compressive trauma to intervertebral discs; walking briskly on grassy ground in the park or on a sandy beach is much kinder to your back. Swimming twice a week is also excellent back exercise.

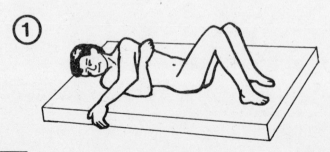

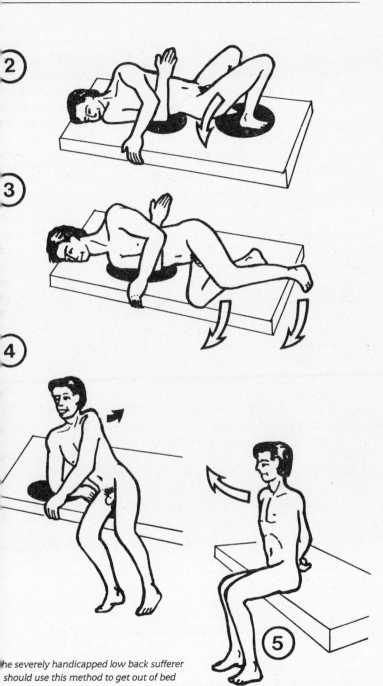

he severely handicapped low back sufferer should use this method to get out of bed

Therapeutic Osteopathic Exercises

Region: Lower back (lumbar) – to improve low back mobilit

Procedure: Stand with knees straight. Raise right heel and stand
the ball of your right foot, while slightly dropping your right should
Return to standing position and repeat on other side.

Action: Perform exercise by alternating movement from side
side. **Note:** DO NOT bend knees during exercise; raise one heel a
time only.

Reduction of lumbar hyperlordosis, lumbosacral an sacrovertebral angles (swayback)

Procedure: Lie on a firm surface facing upwards with your kne
bent and head supported. Place your hands in the small of your back
Action: Press down firmly into your hands, tightening abdomin
muscles. Hold for ten seconds breathing normally. While pressir
into your hands, tilt your pelvis towards you by tightening yo
abdominal muscles and lifting your bottom off the floor slight
While holding this position as above, tilt your pelvis further towar
you by tightening your tummy and holding for ten seconds, the
reverse the effort of lifting your buttocks and relax. Repeat after
short rest.

Stretching of spine extensor muscles and side flexors

Procedure: Stand with your side to the wall, feet together and ar
outstretched with your hand against the wall.

Action: Bring your head and shoulders toward your knees while
the same time lifting your pelvis off the floor. Hold this position for fi
seconds, relax and then repeat.

To stretch the calf muscles (gastrosoleus)

Procedure: Stand with your palms on the wall, fingers pointi
upward and your arms fully outstretched. Place your leg to
stretched behind you as far back as possible, keeping the heel on t
floor and your toes pointing straight ahead. Place your other leg
front with your knee bent.

Action: Gently lean towards the wall by bending your elbo
Note: DO NOT bend the knee of your leg to be stretched.

Stretching of hip and front thigh muscles
Procedure: Place the knee of the leg to be stretched on the floor. Place the foot of the other leg in front of you, pointing straight ahead with the knee bent to about right angles. Clasp hands behind you.
Action: Slowly push your pelvis forwards while gently leaning back your upper body.

Stretching of tensor fascia lata
Procedure: Stand with one side to the wall at arm's length. Place your feet together and your arm outstretched with palm on the wall.
Action: Lean the hip to the wall keeping your arm outstretched. Repeat, changing sides.

Stretching of hamstrings (back thigh muscles) and thigh rotators
Procedure: Sit up on a firm surface keeping your leg to be stretched with the back of the knee touching the floor. Bend the knee of the other leg, pointing the knee to the side. Point your outstretched arms towards the toes of the leg to be stretched.
Action: Attempt to touch your toes with long strokes, varying the position of the foot after a few strokes.

Strengthening of knee extensors (quadriceps)
Accessories: Weight boots, or socks tied together with weights
Procedure: Lie on your back with knees bent over the edge of bed.
Action: Raise your foot until the knee is fully extended. Hold for ten seconds, relax then repeat. Perform without weights initially.

Strengthening of the front thigh muscles
Accessories: Rolled-up towel
Procedure: Lie flat on your back with your head supported. Place the rolled-up towel behind one leg just above the knee.
Action: Lift your foot until your leg is fully straightened, hold for ten seconds, relax then repeat. Repeat, using other leg.

Strengthening of quadriceps and hip flexors
Accessories: Weight boots, or socks tied together with weights
Procedure: Lie flat on your back (supine) with your head supported.
Action: Lift one leg to 50 degrees without bending your knee and try
to hold for ten seconds; relax then repeat, using other leg.

Strengthening of inner thigh muscles
Accessories: Rolled-up towel
Procedure: Lie flat on your back with your head supported. Place
the rolled-up towel between your knees.
Action: Squeeze the towel between your knees while rolling your
feet inwards. Hold for ten seconds. Then relax and repeat.

Strengthening of foot muscles and arches
Accessories: Rolling pin, tennis ball, small paper cuttings
Action: Sitting – firmly roll your foot over bottle or rolling pin.
Sitting – firmly roll your foot over a ball.
Sitting – pick up paper cuttings with your toes.
Standing – stand on the ball of your feet, then relax and repeat.
Sitting on the floor – place the soles of your feet together. Try to make
the largest possible oval shape at the instep. Hold for ten seconds,
then relax and repeat.

6 FEMALE AILMENTS

Many women suffer from back pain during pregnancy, and today many women are understandably wary of taking painkillers for it. The standard medical treatments such as drugs or corsets used for the non-pregnant back-pain sufferer, are out of the question. Prolonged periods of bed-rest suggested by doctors are also very impractical, especially if there are already young children in the household. Registered osteopaths have found that gentle manipulation of the pelvic and low back joints, together with soft-tissue massage, can dramatically reduce the pain caused by carrying the extra weight on the loose ligaments of the spine and pelvis. For first-aid for morning sickness in pregnancy, thoroughly massage the muscles around the fourth and fifth thoracic vertebrae and seek manipulative care from a registered osteopath.

The British School of Osteopathy has a pregnant mother's clinic run by Stephen Sandler, D.O., which offers osteopathic treatment, and advice from a resident midwife. In a survey of the first 100 women at the B.S.O. clinic, 74 per cent had lumbar pain and half of these had suffered back pain before becoming pregnant. In 60 per cent of those who had been pregnant before, the back pain originated from the time of their previous pregnancy.

After confinement, the alignment of the pubic joint at the front of the pelvis is often disordered by the passage of the foetal head past the pubic joint and through the birth canal. The pelvic ligaments stretch and allow the pubic joint to separate for birth. However, they do not always realign correctly afterwards, causing back pain, and a check-up is advisable. Two-thirds of the patients at the B.S.O. first went to the clinic before they were twenty weeks pregnant, proving how easily the body is influenced by pregnancy hormones and the altered posture produced by the presence of a baby.

Osteopathy is not dangerous in pregnancy (in fact during the pregnancy, the spine and pelvis should be carefully kept corrected by a registered osteopath), but it may be advisable to leave treatment until after the first fourteen weeks in cases where there is risk of a miscarriage. Strenuous osteopathic technique, particularly the 'back drop', must be avoided.

At the B.S.O. and in Australia, registered osteopaths focus their efforts on pregnancy mainly because they have little or no control over what happens during birth itself. However, in an article appearing in the *Nursing Mirror*, July 1985, two researchers have found that osteopathic treatment during labour reduces the amount of painkillers women need. The technique used was simply a firm pressure over the lower back at the level of the lumbar vertebrae during contractions, which was released between them. In one study, 81 per cent of the women treated, needed less medication for pain relief. In the United States in particular, osteopathic physicians have full rights to practise obstetrics.

For women or girls who are contemplating strenuous or heavy physical activity, it is advisable to check your menstrual cycle, as nearly 70 per cent of women who experience an acute attack of low back pain for the first time do so within three days of a menstrual period: a reduction of the hormone progesterone at the start of a period coincidentally slightly weakens the ligaments of the spine and pelvis. Women should try to avoid heavy lifting or to be extra careful at this time, as the low back is more vulnerable. For excessively painful periods (dysmenorrhoea) try deep strong pressure (inhibition) at the junction of the sacrum (the triangular bone of the pelvis) and the last lumbar vertebra L5. Using the thumb on one side of the spine of L5 and the index knuckle on the other side, deep steady inhibition may relieve the pain of uterine contractions in seconds. Maintain the pressure vigorously until the cramping stops.

Another trigger point helpful for period pain is on the inside of the lower leg just above the bony prominence (middle malleolus) of the ankle. This point is one finger-width behind and three finger-widths above the middle malleolus of the leg, and deep acupressure here is effective to relieve dysmenorrhoea.

Osteopathic lesions of the spine are a main cause of female ailments. The ninth thoracic vertebra is important for the cervix, and normal mobility of the tenth and eleventh thoracics assists to balance hormonal secretions. The sympathetic nerves influence the ovaries from as high as the fourth thoracic segment of the back, but the main areas are the lower thoracic and upper part of the lower back. Functional technique by a registered osteopath can realign a badly positioned womb, and cranial osteopathy is useful to balance hormone functions. Rebalancing these areas can greatly help with painful periods and pregnancy symptoms.

The use of evening primrose oil for its gamma-linoleic acid content is helpful as a dietary supplement for menstrual difficulties.

When women have a pre-existing low back problem they may find it aggravated by the use of tampons. In this situation it is better to use sanitary towels.

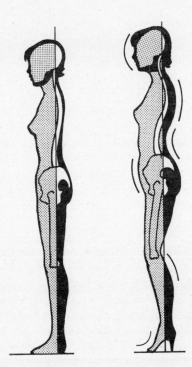

High-heel shoes (as shown on the right) exaggerate normal back curves causing spinal pain. The figure on the left shows normal posture

Fertility and Pregnancy

Old yoga jokes about headstands making you pregnant are no laughing matter to registered osteopaths, who are well aware of the benefits in general of pepping up the blood circulation in the lumbar area. These benefits are also extended to cases of infertility. According to Dr Still, in some cases of sterility, relaxation and correction of the lower thoracics and the upper lumbars 'turns on the uterine artery' increasing the circulation through the reproductive cells. The flow of arterial blood in turn enhances the life and health of the cells, thus making pregnancy possible (unless there is pathological disease), and guards against spontaneous abortion, death of the embryo, deformity of the offspring or defects of the nervous system. The herb raspberry leaf taken as a tea or tablets may assist in the last trimesters.

To have a healthy baby, parents should think well ahead about proper eating. (Books such as Adelle Davis' *Let's Have Healthy Children* are helpful). There is nothing more important for the expectant mother than adequate nutrition. The mother must not starve herself – and her baby – so that she does not gain weight. Professionally prescribed celloid mineral therapy is helpful as an adjunct for infertility and during pregnancy.

As previously mentioned, morning sickness will respond to manipulation of the fifth thoracic vertebra, or it may be due to malposition of the womb due to weakened ligaments in the lower back. Deformities or deficiencies in the newborn can result from osteopathic lesions in the body structures of *either* parent.

Other Causes of Back Pain

One possible cause of back pain which most people overlook is sex. Sexual intercourse can make low back pain much worse if one or the other partner has a pre-existing back lesion and care is not taken. The partner underneath should support the lumbar region with a cushion or pillow. The male partner should not penetrate too deeply as the motion of his hips can strain his back and if he is too vigorous, he can jar his partner's spine and pelvis. The woman should avoid pulling her knees up too far as this can excessively flex the lower back. Sometimes the best position is on the side, so that neither partner has to take the full weight of the other. It is important to be gentle and to not place too great a weight strain on either spine.

Osteopathic Techniques

Although this book gives some ideas for osteopathic first-aid and self-help for the use of any person interested in taking more responsibility for their own life and health, your registered osteopath is a licensed health-care professional who can help you attain a higher level of resistance and immunity to illness and disability. Unlike chiropractors who are restricted to back adjustments of spinal subluxations, osteopathic physicians have a wide range of health-benefiting methods to offer the patient. These are some of the professional techniques or methods used in osteopathic medicine today.

Articulatory technique

A low-velocity gentle manipulation where the dysfunction or lesion of joint motion is engaged repeatedly, or the joint is carried through its entire range of movement in order to increase the freedom of the joint to move easily.

Counterstrain technique

An indirect method developed by an American osteopath, Dr Lawrence Jones. The osteopathic physician moves the part passively away from the area in lesion towards areas of increased motion, always looking for the position of greatest comfort. The osteopathic physician induces a position in the patient of mild, painless strain, based on Jones' idea that the most efficient reflex release occurs when the body is in a position of mild strain in a direction opposite to the lesion. Jones cites a number of trigger points which can be treated for ninety seconds.

Cranial technique

This type of manipulation was discovered by William G. Sutherland, D.O., for treatment applied to the human skull (cranium). Contrary to orthodox opinion, the sutures or joints of the cranium allow very slight movement for fluid circulation through and around the spinal cord and brain.

Direct technique

This is engagement of the lesion directly in the joint and using some method to carry the bone through it. Thrust, high velocity, articulatory and muscle energy are examples of direct manipulation.

Functional technique

This is an indirect method where the osteopathic physician guides the manipulation by feeling at the lesioned part for feedback for comfort of movement. Rather than engaging the osteopathic lesion directly and thrusting through it forcefully, the operator uses gentle mobilisation to find the position of greatest ease and this is followed carefully until joint normality is restored.

High velocity-low amplitude technique

This is the osteopathic method which has been borrowed by most chiropractors. It uses a direct thrust against the barrier of the osteopathic lesion to decisively restore the full range of movement to the part. This is the most dramatic technique as it is used by a large number of osteopaths and others, and the correction is often remembered because of the 'click', 'crunch' or 'pop' that accompanies the separation of the surfaces of the joint capsule. Because it is an aggressive method and potentially dangerous, it should never be attempted by the layperson, although it is quite safe in the hands of the fully qualified doctor of osteopathy.

Indirect technique

A manipulative technique where the motion barrier in the joint is disengaged. The lesioned bone or part is moved away from the motion barrier to a point of simultaneous balance and decreased tension. This includes functional technique and counterstrain technique.

Inhibition

The application of steady pressure to soft tissues to cause relaxation and normalise reflexes.

Muscle energy technique

This term was first suggested by Fred Mitchell Snr, D.O., to describe osteopathic manipulative therapy (O.M.T.) where the patient uses his or her muscles, on request from the doctor of osteopathy, from a position on the motion barrier, against a precisely executed counterforce offered by the doctor. (The motion barrier is that section of the lesioned joint surface that is jammed or restricted and unable to move freely.) This is an isometric manipulation where the reflex effect of the voluntary muscle effort of the patient in a precisely controlled position against the operator resistance, resolves the joint barrier.

Soft-tissue technique

This is outlined in other chapters, but it is essentially manipulation of the soft parts of the body other than the skeleton, using stretching, drainage, deep pressure, traction, and separation of the muscle origin and insertion. It is also known as neuromuscular technique.

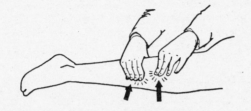

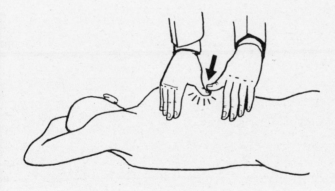

This is soft tissue technique, or neuromuscular massage,
as used on the back and legs

7 USEFUL EXERCISES

Nature has a way of maintaining good muscle tone and flexibility by stretching. Watch a cat or dog after they have been resting; the first thing they do is stretch. Animals stretch by habit, and Nature maintains flexibility of joints, muscles and ligaments this way so that after any inactivity, stretching is done to loosen tight muscles and ligaments.

Stretching does several things – connective tissue shortens when not stretched, and stiffening occurs. Stretching lengthens them and allows muscles to relax. Stretching relaxes and limbers up the large muscles and ligaments, thus making the body more flexible.

Bad posture can overstrain the muscles and ligaments. Age can cause this condition also. As you grow older, muscles become shorter and tighter (especially when not in use) and lose tone. Inactivity can cause the same problem. A tightened or contracted muscle or ligament also reduces the range of motion of the facet joints of the back, making them prone to jamming up or becoming hypomobile. This in turn causes an osteopathic lesion in the spine, interfering with the expression of nerve supply to the muscles and organs. Any cases of ill-health can be traced to these structural problems by your osteopathic physician. (Be sure that your osteopathic practitioner is fully registered or licensed in the State or country where you live.)

Therapeutic Osteopathic Exercise

When to exercise – the time to exercise is right now or at any time. During the day, be exercise- and posture-conscious. Only seconds are required to take a few deep breaths, stretch, correct your posture, or contract a group of muscles. Taking an exercise break for just a few seconds or minutes will improve your efficiency and health. Exercise in the morning by stretching to loosen up muscles and ligaments; during the day for better posture, better breathing, and take deep breaths for alertness and general toning up; in the evening to help fatigued muscles and to restore better circulation.

Develop a regular exercise period for ten minutes each day at your convenience. That is all that's needed for general spinal conditioning. It is advisable to have a thorough osteopathic examination prior to starting your exercise programme.

Exercise on a comfortable surface. It is best to do exercises prescribed by your registered osteopath. Avoid 'weekend only' sport, as rigorous activity only once a week will serve only to overstress the spine and body in general. If you are in a sedentary occupation and your job involves much sitting or stooping for long periods, pause frequently to walk around for a few minutes.

Caution Concerning Exercise

Too many people become discouraged with exercising because they overdo the first day, leaving themselves stiff and sore, even to the point of straining their vertebrae (osteopathic lesions), so that they are reluctant to try it again. So, if you are beginning your exercises for the first time, quit before you get too fatigued. If you have discontinued exercise for some time, start from the beginning; do less than you were doing when you stopped.

If you are stiff from exercise the day before, cut back the number of exercises. Never force a stiff muscle – you can injure it. Work at it gradually, using more stretching exercises.

Spinal exercises cannot correct postural deficiencies which are congenital in origin. Neither will they correct spinal misalignments. When corrective manipulation is given to fix an osteopathic lesion and the cause of the particular health problem is removed or eased, these specific exercises will help in maintaining improved health by improving spinal stability. If any prescribed exercise causes pain either during or after its performance, discontinue that activity and consult your registered osteopath.

Region: Neck (cervical vertebrae)
General mobility – stretching of the flexor and extensor muscles
Procedure: Sit comfortably with back straight. Fix eyes on an object at eye level in the distance.

Action: While looking at the object thrust head forward and backward.

Caution: Perform slowly. If any discomfort is experienced, pain, dizziness, etc. DO NOT continue and contact your registered osteopath.

General mobility – stretching of neck side flexor muscles
Procedure: Sit comfortably, keeping head upright. Take head to right side (right ear to right shoulder). Place right hand over your head with fingers just above your left ear.

Action: Using your right hand gently pull your head towards the right side in stretching fashion. Relax and repeat on the left side using your left hand.

General mobility of neck
Procedure: Sit comfortably with back straight. Turn your head towards the left. Raise your right elbow to eye level and place right hand over your right temple with fingers pointing to the front and thumb to the rear (with your palm over your ear).
Action: Gently push your head to a maximum painfree rotation in a stretching fashion. Relax and repeat the exercise on the opposite side of the head using your left hand.

General mobility – stretching of neck flexor muscles
Procedure: Sit comfortably with back straight. Take your head and shoulders back to a comfortable maximum.
Action: Gently rock your head backwards.
Caution: Perform this slowly. If any discomfort is experienced, pain or dizziness, DO NOT continue and consult your registered osteopath.

General mobility – stretching of extensor muscles
Procedure: Take your head to a comfortable maximum in the forward direction. (DO NOT continue if any discomfort is experienced.) If no discomfort is experienced, interlock your fingers behind your head, above the top of your neck.
Action: Using your hands, stretch your head forward gently.
Caution: Perform slowly. If any discomfort is experienced DO NOT continue and consult your registered osteopath.

Stretching of neck extensor muscles and reduction of neck hyperlordosis
Accessories: Rolled-up towel, two pillows
Procedure: Lie down on your back on a firm surface. Place two pillows under your head. Place rolled-up towel under spine and shoulders. Tuck your chin in and push your head against the pillows very gently.

Region: Shoulder and arm (upper extremities)
Stretching of wrist extensor muscles (forearm muscles)
Procedure: Place your arm directly in front of you, with your elbow locked straight and your palm facing down. Bend your wrist down in the direction of your palm.
Action: Using your other hand, grasp the back of your hand of the outstretched arm and pull it towards you, causing the wrist to bend slightly further. You should be able to feel your forearm muscles being stretched. Continue rhythmical stretching action, while slowly moving your hand down and back to level position. The wrist flexor muscles can also be stretched by extending your arm as above but with your wrist bent up in the direction of the back of your hand, with other hand grasping palmar side of fingers. Proceed with the action described above. These moves are beneficial for R.S.I. sufferers.

General stretching of shoulder joint capsules
Accessories: Stool, moderate weight (such as an old iron)
Procedure: Bend your trunk forward at the waist approximately at right angles, supporting your body with one hand on a high stool or firm shelf. Let your other arm hang down while holding the weight.
Action: Swing the weight-bearing arm from front to back, slowly increasing the range. Swing the arm from side to side slowly increasing the range. Swing the arm in a circular motion, at the side of your body, forming increasingly larger circles in a clockwise direction. Repeat in an anticlockwise direction.

Stretching of shoulder capsule
Procedure: Stand facing the wall with your arm with the affected shoulder outstretched in front of you, and the index and middle fingers touching the wall.
Action: Cause the fingers to climb the wall while slowly turning your body until you are facing side-on to the wall – it does not matter whether you turn your body into your shoulder or away from it.

Stretching of the front shoulder capsule and pectoral muscles
Procedure: Stand facing the corner between walls, arms bent at waist level and palms on the walls.
Action: Push forward into the corner then away from it. Move your hands a little further up the wall after each push up. Repeat until your arms are fully elevated.

Caution: Avoid arching your back and neck.

To increase shoulder joint mobility with general stretching of shoulder capsule

Procedure: Sit with elbows elevated and slightly forwards, with your hands next to your ears.

Action: Roll your elbows up, back and downwards in a circular fashion, coming back to your starting position.

Region: Rib cage and spine (thoracics)
To reduce neck and upper back stoop

Procedure: Stand with knees straight and hips bent forwards at right angles. Clasp your hands behind your back, keeping elbows straight.

Action: Arch your back whilst lifting your head, hands, and pulling your shoulder blades together. Hold for five seconds then relax completely, dropping your head and arms for five seconds. Repeat up to three minutes, alternating action and relaxation.

Note: This exercise can also be performed sitting on a stool.

To stretch rib cage and pectoral muscles, increase rib expansion and reduce 'humpback' (kyphosis)

Procedure: Stand in a relaxed position, arms at the side.

Action: Breathe in deeply while elevating arms above head; then lean back gently, looking at hands. Slowly return head to level position and bring your arms down to relaxed position, breathing out fully. Repeat four or five times.

To stretch rib cage, improve expansion and reduce kyphosis

Procedure: Stand comfortably with arms outstretched forwards.

Action: Breathe in deeply while bringing arms backwards. While holding a full breath, fold palms upwards and gently push further backwards. Slowly bring your arms down to a relaxed position, while breathing out fully. Repeat four or five times.

To improve kyphosis and to stretch thoracic muscles

Procedure: Stand or sit with your back and head straight. Place your hands against the breast bone (sternum) in prayer position.

Action: Breathe in deeply while pressing chest into your hands, by slowly bringing your shoulders and elbows forwards. Hold briefly and slowly breathe out.

Walking is one of the most natural things you can do and therefore it is a healthy exercise for all ages. It gives you mobility, muscular coordination and aids natural body functions. Walking is a good total body exercise, tones muscles, burns off excess fat and induces proper breathing. Brisk walking is better exercise than jogging because it improves cardiovascular blood supply without the high-impact trauma on your discs and hip joints of pounding the pavements.

'Inversion equipment' has become very popular to relieve low back and joint pain by hanging upside down in hooked boots from a door lintel or in a metal frame. This treatment might help relieve pressure of a narrowed or herniated intervertebral disc. It is certainly easier on the vertebrae of the upper neck than yoga headstands. However, for older patients it does have an element of risk, particularly if there is a history of high blood pressure and the risk of a stroke or bursting of the blood vessels in the brain – the body has many subtle mechanisms for pumping fluid out of the legs and keeping blood up to the head. Also, research at the Chicago College of Osteopathic Medicine has implicated hanging suspended for any length of time by inversion boots, with an increase of fluid pressure in the eyeball (intraocular pressure). This is not good news if you have glaucoma or a family history of this disease, which can lead progressively to blindness. Consult a physician or registered osteopath before attempting any inversion exercise.

8 SOFT-TISSUE MASSAGE

The role of soft tissue in the human body in health and disease deserves attention. The muscles, connective tissues and fascia (which surround the muscles) are vital to the total economy of the body. The nutrition, nerve supply and drainage of each part of the body is essential and the many ways that osteopathic lesions in the soft tissues reflect deeper disease of both body and mind through nerve reflex, are also important. If the blood and lymph are denied easy access to cells they bathe, the exchange of oxygen, cell foods and waste by-products is cut back and the tissues become susceptible to disease.

There are many systems for treatment of nerve and body reflexes including foot zone therapy, Chapman's reflexes, muscle-fascia trigger points (developed by Dr Janet Travell and used by osteopathic physicians) and Chinese acupuncture – and the common factor is that they are found in fascia tissue around the muscles.

Fascia is a fibrous membrane around muscles (the word comes from the same Latin word as 'Fascist', for the bundles of sticks and axes that symbolised Roman political power). Stresses and strains in fascia produce definite patterns, related to lines of postural stress, which are found in all patients. Andrew Taylor Still said the fascia is the place to look for the causes of disease and the place to begin the action of remedies.

Restrictions of joint mobility, postural distortions of body alignment, and muscle spasms are important, not because of local pain and discomfort, but because of reflex effect on other body areas. Tender areas of spasm – felt or palpated by your osteopathic physician – are more significant than just back pain, joint sprains and muscle injuries, and can be measured scientifically by changes of electrical potential of the skin.

Osteopathic soft-tissue or muscle massage is known in Britain as neuromuscular technique (N.M.T.) and in Australia as kinetic tissue manipulation. It is widely believed that osteopathy consists of manipulation suitable only for the relief of joint strains of the spine. Osteopathy is, however, much broader in its application, and the purely mechanical myth is dispelled by its use for soft tissues.

The responsibility for developing neuromuscular technique is originally credited to the South African Stanley Lief, who was born in Latvia, in the Baltic, in the 1890s. The Lief family emigrated to South Africa in the 1900s and both Leon Chaitow, who has written on osteopathy, and Brian Wilson, who co-founded the New Zealand Register of Osteopaths, are related to Stanley Lief, called the father of British Nature Cure.

Lief qualified in osteopathy in the U.S.A. some time before 1914. In 1925 he founded his health farm, Champneys, at Tring in England, and at this world-famous health centre he established a reputation as a daring and pioneering osteopathic physician, developing a huge following. During his most successful years before the second world war, he evolved soft-tissue technique, described by his nephew Leon Chaitow, D.O., in his book: *Neuro-Muscular Technique – A Practitioner's Guide to Soft-Tissue Manipulation,* (Thorsons).

The modality of neuromuscular technique may be studied from Chaitow's book and incorporated into any system of physical medicine. It is most useful as a precedent of manipulative therapy and its use has been literally in the hands of the osteopathic profession. It has been cited as the distinctive feature of osteopathic manipulation to distinguish it from chiropractic which, in practice, ignores soft tissue. Andrew Taylor Still introduced the 'Rule of the Artery' to emphasise the dependence of muscle freedom for blood flow for the internal organs.

However, the soft tissue part of musculoskeletal dysfunction (or osteopathic lesion) of the body is the source of a great deal of pain and disease, whether local or general or by nerve reflex, or referred in origin.

Such diagnostic terms as 'fibrositis' or 'muscular rheumatism' used by doctors, although popular, do not indicate anything scientifically. For accuracy, the definition given by the prestigious American Academy of Osteopathy and adopted by the World Health Organisation as part of the International Classification of Diseases, can be applied to lesions or dysfunction of the musculoskeletal system: 'Somatic dysfunction or, as defined, impaired or altered function of related components of the somatic [body framework] system, i.e. skeletal, arthrodial [of the joints] and myofascial [muscles and their fasciae] structures and related vascular, lymphatic and nerve elements'.

Sixty per cent of the body mass comprises the musculoskeletal system and as well as being our structural framework, it is the main consumer of body energy. Apart from the obvious role of support and movement of the body, it has biochemical and biomechanical activities. Ida Rolf, Ph.D., whose massage 'rolfing' system was popular with the human potential movement in California during the 1970s, suggested humans were an energy mass subject to gravity.

As the osteopathic profession grew in Australia from its humble beginnings in 1959, neuromuscular methods were increasingly used as kinetic tissue manipulation. Wallace C. Brown, D.O., described the theory of his methods as follows:

'People today little realise that when they push or stroke their forehead with the palm of their hand during headache, fatigue or stress they are probably engaging in one of many natural reactions which no doubt formed the foundation of manipulative therapy dating as far back as man himself.

'To the layman osteopathic kinetic tissue manipulation is probably more broadly associated with the term "massage"; and although the osteopathic approach includes some applications similar to massage, its therapy is much deeper and more detailed and is primarily directed toward reduction of the immobile joint. Nextly, it is concerned with peripheral pressure and congestion of organs, nerve, blood and lymph created by local-zone spasms and it's this latter form of kinetic tissue manipulation that only in some respects and in some cases resembles the massage that is commonly practised today...

'Medical physiotherapy today follows along the line of Lucas-Championniere of France and this is the more gentle form of massage. The deeper kinetic tissue manipulation of the osteopath would appear to be unknown to modern medical practice.'

Osteopathic Massage

Osteopathic massage or muscle manipulation is peculiar to osteopathy and is used by registered osteopaths as one method to correct muscle lesions associated with bone-joint misalignments in the body. Other methods developed and utilised by osteopathic physicians include fascial unwinding, muscle energy technique, strain-counterstrain and functional release. Applied kinesiology is another way of treating muscle imbalance that was discovered by chiropractors and used by chiropractors and osteopaths. These are professional methods, but one treatment which can be safely used by the layperson is deep-tissue massage.

Osteopathic massage is not to be confused with massage in the accepted and practical use of the term. Physiotherapy and Swedish massage in the accepted or ordinary practice of medicine is used to relieve pain temporarily by attempting to bring muscles to tone and flexibility without tenderness or conscious restriction. As applied

medically, massage refers to relief of minor disabilities and is consist
ent with its limited concept. Its method is superficial by comparison
with the work of the registered osteopath, and massage is aimed a
promoting a feeling of muscular well-being.

Osteopathic soft-tissue work, on the other hand, is directed to th
osteopathic lesion and that implies spastic, fibritic sustained contrac
tion or contracture, usually of the muscles within 25 mm of either sid
of the spine (spinous processes) called the paravertebrals. Persisten
toughness of these muscles and fascia both residual and 'acute' o
pain, is always associated with a locking or hypomobility of the joint
of the back.

Although relief in some acute and chronic spinal lesions of the bacl
is sometimes effected without attending to the muscle tissues as ir
chiropractic adjustment, results for the patient will be very mucl
more limited. Osteopathy, however, is holistic in approach to th
body and considers it incomplete to leave muscle lesions uncorrected
and because of its philosophy, osteopathy often assists cases whicl
have not responded to chiropractic or other therapies, and the result
of osteopathic treatment likewise are more lasting. The use of variou
parts of the arms, besides the hands, for the purpose of deep-tissue
massage, is essential for gentle penetration of the muscle layers of the
body and the necessary muscle give and release of the tissues an
fascia.

The uniqueness of osteopathic contact points has been frownec
upon as too severe, but rolfing is one method that has been borrowec
from osteopathy (its namesake, Ida Rolf, formulated her ideas while
teaching at the Philadelphia College of Osteopathic Medicine).*

Skill of a high order is necessary to manipulate muscles osteo
pathically and it is a serious study not to be treated lightly by student
in eagerness to arrive at other manipulative techniques. However, i
used conservatively and thoughtfully it can be responsibly used by
the non-professional as first-aid for back pain until you can get the
patient to a registered osteopath.

Usually the osteopath's hands would be applied directly to the
patient's skin, using a suitable natural massage oil. Always be carefu
that your hands are warm. Contacts with the skin should be made
gently but firmly. Rhythm should tend to be too slow rather than too
rapid. Rapid movement on the body is directly stimulating and
psychologically, may cause the patient to think that the masseur i
hurried and disinterested.

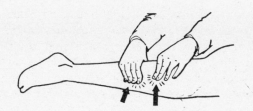

Drainage of the calf muscle

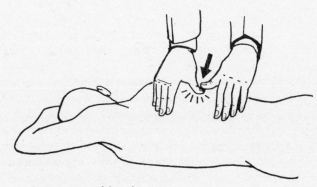

Deep massage of the spine.
The area should be to within 25 mm of the bones

When an osteopathic lesion of the joint articulation occurs, the surrounding muscles are briefly relaxed at first, but at once pass into contraction to naturally splint the back. This interferes with the easy correction of the lesion as well as drainage of waste fluids such as venous blood and lymph from the part. If the osteopathic lesion persists, the muscles may go into permanent contracture, with later production of fibrous tissues and, at the end, atrophy of the muscle.

Active exercise of muscles produces acidosis, and heat applied to the body tissues induces alkalosis. Soft-tissue manipulation and massage has neither of these effects, but does induce an increased percentage of haemoglobin and red blood cell count (erythrocyte). It also produces a tonic effect on the metabolism, both in the local part and the whole body, due to an effect on the small arteries and capillaries. Manipulation of the soft tissues is one of the useful measures known to present-day therapeutics.

Osteopathy is not a glorified form of massage, and correction of soft tissue lesions is important. It is preparatory to the correction of bony lesions to the end that adjustment may be made with a minimum of effort and trauma by the registered osteopath. After soft-tissue work, osteopathic manipulation inflicts no trauma to the patient and there is a greater likelihood that the correction will be maintained.

The two most effective methods of relaxing muscle tissue are (a) to press at right angles to the muscle fibres and (b) to stretch by separating the origin and insertion of the muscle.‡ Pressure duration for sustained inhibition of muscle fibres is in the vicinity of four second of pressure with two seconds off; up to thirty seconds on with thirty seconds off. Elbows, knuckles, fingers, forearm are all useful as contact points, along with the palms and pads of the fingers and thumbs, and their use is dependent on each patient. Reaction firstly of the patient and secondly of the tissue, is the best guide to being overenthusiastic in applying deep-tissue massage.

For many years registered osteopaths have reported that O.M.T. is beneficial for mental and emotional problems. Recently medical doctors at Bangor Hospital in the U.K. investigated the effects of connective-tissue massage on patients suffering from mental tension and anxiety. Psychophysiological tests were taken before and after connective-tissue massage (which resembles osteopathic muscle manipulation). All the patients showed a significant response to massage treatment on one or more of the tests. The group of patients chosen for the trial had impaired circulation, muscular tension, pain and sleep disturbances. Patients talked about sensations of warmth and a feeling of tranquillity, and frequently reported deep refreshing sleep following treatment with massage. A consistent and important finding by the doctors was that as the physical tension was unlocked, so the patients began to talk at length and with appropriate emotion about their emotional or psychological problem. As their body armour was broken down, they relived the origins of their emotional and mental problems.

* Rolfing uses the same deep-tissue contact points to release emotional and physical trauma locked into the soft tissues and muscles. An emotional catharsis often follows effective deep body manipulation and realignment.

‡ The origin and insertion of a muscle are the points where that muscle is attached to bone by tendons and mechanical leverage can effectively stretch a muscle if the respective attachments are further separated by gentle manipulation.

9 OSTEOPATHIC FIRST-AID

General Soft-Tissue Technique

● Example: the front surface of the right thigh. With the patient supine, the masseur stands at the right side of the massage table opposite the patient's thigh. With hands slightly cupped, the palms are placed against the surface of the leg. As the masseur applies pressure, he visualises the muscles being pressed gently against the patient's femur or upper leg bone. The hands are rolled away from the operator; released; reapplied. A rhythmical procedure should be developed.

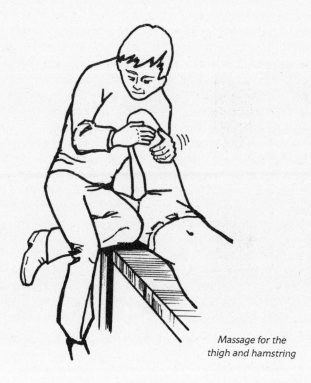

Massage for the thigh and hamstring

● With the masseur and the patient in the same position, the muscles are then grasped between finger tips and palm, producing gentle pressure followed by a careful lifting to slightly separate muscle away from the femur. Great care should be taken not to apply too much force – and to press, does not mean to pinch.

Drainage of the calf muscles

This treatment is excellent first-aid for a strained or swollen ankle.

- The patient should be supine, while the masseur sits on the edge of the treatment table opposite the patient's knee, facing the head of the table. The patient's knee is flexed to a right angle and the calf of the leg is grasped with both hands so that the thumbs are over the tibia and the fingers are touching over the calf muscle (gastrocnemius). While compressing the calf, the tissues and fluids are gently pumped towards the knee; the grip is then relaxed. This is repeated several times. The manoeuvre must be done slowly and gently, the fingers describing a small circle, to produce lymphatic drainage.

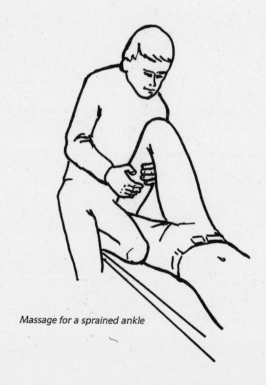

Massage for a sprained ankle

● The patient's leg is placed over the operator's nearest shoulder, the proximal part of the thigh is grasped with both hands. The thigh muscles are slowly but firmly rotated clockwise around the femur, and pressed towards the pelvis. The grip is relaxed and the manoeuvre repeated several times, each time the hands being placed about 30 mm nearer the knee. Clockwise and counterclockwise rotations are alternated. Upon reaching the knee, the manipulation of the calf is repeated.

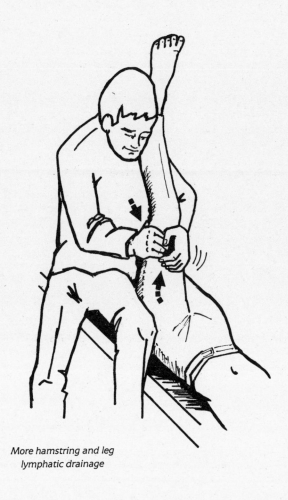

*More hamstring and leg
lymphatic drainage*

Manipulation of the soft tissues of the back

Relaxation of the muscles of the back may be accomplished by applying deep pressure at right angles to the longitudinal direction of the muscles, and over their attachments. The student of osteopathy should learn to palpate while doing soft-tissue work.

• The patient lies on his side. Facing him, the masseur semiflexes the index finger of his hand, completely flexing his other fingers. Placing the fleshy portion of the fingertips in contact with the skin of the patient's back just above the line of the spinal bones (spinous processes), he exerts pressure on the back muscles, accompanied by a slight sideways pull of the fingertips. He then releases the pressure. The manoeuvre is repeated at intervals throughout the thoracic and low back area. The work should be done slowly.

• The patient then lies prone on the treatment table. Standing at the side, the masseur places the thumb of one hand parallel with and adjacent to the spine (spinous processes) on the far side. The thumb is reinforced with the palm of the opposite hand. With firm pressure towards the table, the masseur slightly rotates both hands counter-clockwise and then clockwise, or rolls his thumbs away from the spine. This is repeated at intervals throughout the lower back and thoracic areas. Care must be taken to avoid slipping your thumb on the patient's skin or pulling soft tissues over the bony prominences of the back, as both are painful and bruising. The work should be done slowly, and is repeated on the opposite side.

• The patient again lies on his side. Facing him, the masseur places his forearm against the crest of the hip bone (ilium) and his other forearm against the armpit (axilla). His hands are side by side, with fingertips applied to the back muscles above the spine. Gently, but firmly, he pulls the muscle away from the spine and towards himself. This manoeuvre is particularly good in the lower back (lumbar) and lower chest (thoracic) areas, and is used advantageously on thin or sensitive patients.

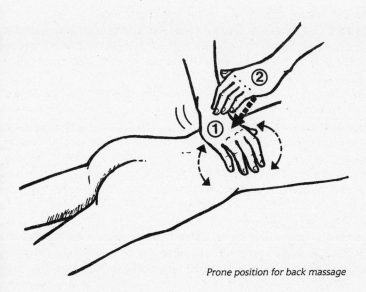

Prone position for back massage

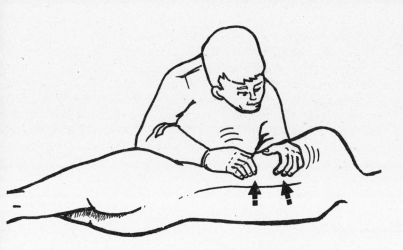

Side-lying spinal massage

Manipulation of the soft tissues of the neck

Manipulation of the neck SHOULD NEVER be attempted by any person not professionally qualified in osteopathy, as death can result from injury of the vertebral artery, particularly if the neck is in extension at the time. Contraindications include cholesterol plaque or hardening of the artery which runs through the neck vertebrae to deliver blood to the base of the brain. Only a registered osteopath is fully trained to test and diagnose the cervical area to prevent such a disaster.

If the patient experiences any pain, dizziness, faint or any symptoms during neck exercise or soft-tissue massage or stretching, STOP THE MOVEMENT at once and consult a registered osteopath.

• The patient lies supine. Standing at the side of the treatment table, the masseur places his hand on the patient's forehead and his other hand on the far side of the neck, keeping the tips of his fingers sideways to the spine. The masseur pulls towards himself with one hand while his closer hand rotates the patient's head in the same direction, but maintains resistance. If the patient complains of dizziness, hold the head in the midline, avoiding rotation in either direction.

• After having relaxed the neck muscles, the masseur places his right forearm under the patient's neck and grasps the left shoulder with his fingers. Placing his left hand on the forehead, he alternately raises and lowers his right forearm while the head is being rotated with the left hand. The procedure is repeated on the opposite side.

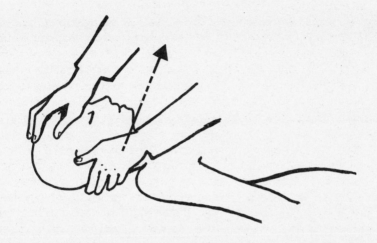

Do not continue if distress is caused

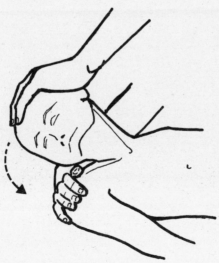

Gentle stretches of the neck

● Then the patient lies supine. The masseur stands at the end of the treatment table and grasps the base of the head (occiput) with his right hand. Placing the left hand on the patient's right shoulder, he passes his forearm under the patient's neck. Slowly the cervical spine is side-bent and rotated towards the left, then towards the right, until the right ear is close to the right shoulder. The position of the hands is reversed and the manoeuvre is repeated on the left side. The hand on the base of the head may add a moderate amount of gentle rotation if desired. The masseur now crosses his forearms under the patient's head, and places his hands on opposite shoulders. By changing position of the masseur's body, the patient's neck may be flexed gently, side-bent and rotated.

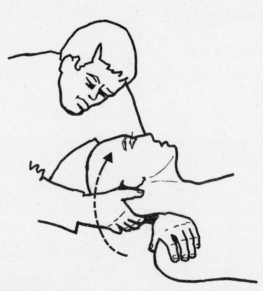

*Side-bending stretch
of the neck vertebrae*

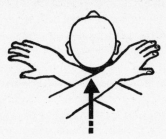

Arm position for neck stretching

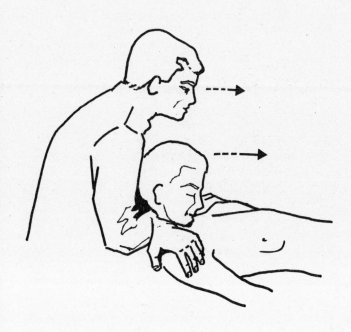

Care should be taken to avoid patient distress

Manipulation of the soft tissue of the arms

● The masseur places his forearm under the patient's arm, allowing the latter's forearm to hang loosely over the operator's arm. The fingers of his hand grasp the inside edge (medial margin) of the shoulder blade (scapula), and the masseur's other hand is placed over the deltoid muscle of the patient's arm. The patient's shoulder may now be rotated, thereby stretching the muscles attached to the shoulder blade.

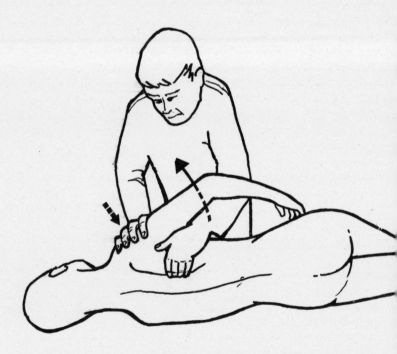

Gentle stretch for a strained shoulder

Osteopathic First-Aid for Common Ailments

Wryneck (or torticollis) is a painful unnatural spasm of one side of the muscles of the neck causing the head to be drawn to one side. Until the patient can be taken to see a registered osteopath, the use of Chapman's reflexes for wryneck is valuable first-aid for this condition. Chapman's reflexes are a system of trigger points taught also in the 'Touch for Health' system as neurolymphatic points. Refer to the illustration below.

According to Frank Chapman, D.O., a contraction at the inner aspect of the upper end of the bone of the arm (humerus) from just below the ball-and-socket joint (surgical neck) downwards is indicative of wryneck. The other points to treat are at the back of the side protuberances (transverse processes) of the third, fourth, sixth and seventh neck vertebrae.

The amount of soreness of the points at the front of the arm will indicate the extent of lymphatic blockage of fluids in the neck muscles, and gentle massage there will relieve soreness in the neck. This will render neck treatment by your registered osteopath more tolerant to the patient.

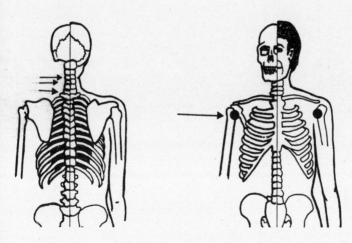

Treatment points for torticollis

Sinusitis

Reflex centres to relieve sinus pain that may have continued fc
weeks, will be found in the ribs and on the back of the second nec
(cervical) vertebra. At the front of the body a ropy contraction will b
felt about 90 mm from the breastbone (sternum) on the upper edg
of the second rib and in the muscle above.

The point in the neck is midway between the spine of C2 and th
tip of the side protuberance (transverse process). A complete rela
ation of both reflex centres will relieve the sinus patient, but th
patient should attend a registered osteopath for cranial osteopathy t
release any misplacement in the sutures of the head, and allow drair
age of the sinuses. Diet should also be attended to. Refer to the illu
tration opposite.

Sciatica

At the front of the body, ropy contractions indicating lymphat
congestion associated with nerve pain running down one or bot
legs, will be found at a number of reflex centres:

• A ropy point starting one-fifth of the distance below the larg
bony protuberance of the femur (bone of the upper leg), known a
the trochanter, and for a space of 50 to 90 mm downwards on th
back outer aspect of the femur.

• A ropy point commencing one-fifth of the distance above th
knee and continuing upward for a matter of 50 mm on the back oute
aspect of the bone of the upper leg.

• A ropy point in the mid-back region of the femur and one-thir
of the distance upward from the joints of the knee (condyles).

Dr Chapman called this ropiness a 'gangliform contraction' in th
fascia and claimed that a considerable amount of soreness at all thre
regions indicated sciatic neuritis. He also suggested the followin
supplemental points:

• Both sides of the outer bone of the lower leg (fibula) from i
upper attachment or articulation with the large bone of the lower le
(tibia) to the outer rounded protuberance (malleolus).

• Midway between the large protuberance of the femu
(trochanter) across the muscles just above the femur and the pelvis

- Just below the back of the large edge of the pelvis.

The main point of the reflex centres at the back of the patient is on the upper part of the triangular bone at the base of the spine (sacrum) just inside its joint to the pelvic bones (sacroiliac joint). An innominate *fn) lesion (of the sacroiliac joints) will be found, and the patient should have manipulation of the lower spine by a registered osteopath as soon as possible after these reflex points have been treated by massage. Refer to the illustration below.

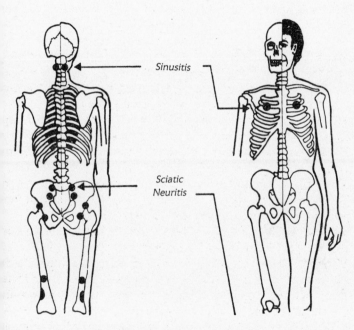

Sinusitis

Sciatic Neuritis

First-aid points for sinusitis and sciatica

* The innominate bone is the large bone of the hip joint comprising the ilium, ischium and pubis.

Atonic constipation

The Chapman's reflex to relieve constipation will be found in th
muscle tissue between the front lip of the pelvic bone (the anteri
superior spine of the ilium) and the side protuberance of the upper le
bone (femur). Ropiness here indicates loss of tone of the large inte
tine with dilation and constipation.

At the back, the reflex will be found on the face of the eleventh ri
at the end of the side protuberance (transverse process) of th
eleventh thoracic vertebra in the rib cage area. Attention should als
be given to the diet to ensure that there is sufficient fibre and that
natural diet of fresh vegetables and fruit is followed. Refer to the illu
tration on page below.

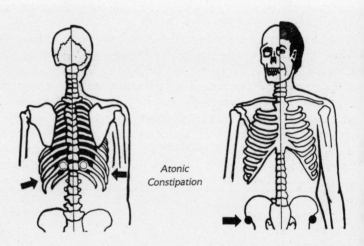

Atonic
Constipation

Treatment points for constipation

Laryngitis

The Chapman's reflex for huskiness or loss of voice with attendant cough, is found at the front of the rib cage on the upper surface of the second rib, from 50 to 90 mm from the breastbone. At the back of the neck a reflex point will be found midway between the tip of the side of the second neck vertebra C2, and the spine of the vertebra (spinous process).

Abdominal massage

A special use of neuromuscular technique by Stanley Lief, D.O., was the treatment of deep-seated adhesions, contractions and muscle spasms in the abdominal area, particularly where the stomach muscles were a source of pain and discomfort after a surgical operation. Lief's method of breaking up stomach adhesions become known as 'bloodless surgery'.

Chaitow describes them as abdominal release, stating: 'These "release" techniques can be applied to soft areas of the body (e.g. the throat) as well as to the abdomen. The original concept of "bloodless surgery" was that adhesions were being "peeled" away from their anchorage by the technique and in some cases this might have been so. However, its application is to any area of tight, fibrosed, spastic, contracted or adhering soft tissue in the abdominal region. The most dramatic improvements in function are noted after its use in such conditions as spastic or atonic constipation, visceroptosis, dysmenorrhoea, and menorrhagia, as well as ill-defined abdominal congestion and pain.

'Precisely what takes place after release technique is open to conjecture. An improvement in tone and circulation, and usually general function, is the most obvious result. It is a matter of debate whether this is because of a release of the long-held contractive state in the soft tissues or because of an actual breaking of adhesions or because of some other mechanism.'

Stanley Lief applied his abdominal massage to release post-operative adhesions, under subdued red light, to induce as deep a relaxation as possible.

Collagen Fibres

Collagen is the protein substance found in the connective tissues of the body, concerned with supporting the organs and parts and binding them together. The fascia are used for food storage and as part of the body defence mechanisms, moving about and neutralising cell toxins as well as regulating mineral (electrolyte) balance.

Most people today are aware of diet and nutrition and its role in the defence of the body, and many practitioners have held that many collagen diseases, such as rheumatoid arthritis, have a nutritional cause. Modern research has increasingly pointed to the protective effects of nutrients such as Vitamin C on joint surfaces and soft tissues in general.

The functional efficiency of connective tissues, according to British osteopath Brian K. Youngs, D.O., particularly is important to the structural integrity of the spine. Youngs points to cases of chronic back pain where the so-called 'Black Line Phenomenon' has suggested an underlying nutritional deficiency. British osteopaths using a spinal meter (to detect the electrical potential of the skin over the most active osteopathic lesions), have commonly found that pressure 5 mm on each side of the spine by a probe will illicit a dark blue or black line. The pressure of the hemispherical probe is very light as it is intended to register variations in skin resistance, but it has an effect on the small arteries and veins of the capillary network under the skin surface. Swelling of the capillaries with blue venous blood causes the appearance of the black line which slowly fades as the impeded circulation returns to the local skin.

It was another British practitioner, Keither Lamont, D.O., who drew attention to the fact that administration of Vitamin E, bioflavinoid complex and potentised iron phosphate will correct the deficiency associated with Black Line Phenomenon. Lamont suggested a co-existing blood anomaly with either low haemoglobin or low serum iron levels in patients.

The popular view of osteopathy is that it is only concerned with adjusting displaced vertebrae or relieving trapped nerves by a simple manipulation. While this may frequently and effectively work, the fact that some people regularly have a 'bone put back' indicates that unqualified manipulation is only temporary. A fully-qualified osteopath will attend to the 'whole patient' for the causes of disease.

10 WHERE TO FIND A REGISTERED OSTEOPATH

The addresses below are of properly qualified osteopathic physicians and recognised osteopathic associations and colleges where further information about and directories of the osteopathic profession can be readily obtained.

UNITED KINGDOM
Birmingham & District Osteopathic Clinic
955 Stratford Road, Hall Green, Birmingham 28
Ph (021) 777 5757

Sheffield Osteopathic Practitioners' Clinic
Victoria Hall (Chapel Walk Entrance), Norfolk Street, Sheffield 1
Ph 0742 53774

The General Council and Register of Osteopaths
21 Suffolk Street, London S.W.1
Ph (01) 839 2060

The British Naturopathic and Osteopathic Association
Fraser House, 6 Netherhall Gardens, London
Ph (01) 435 7830

The Osteopathic Association
8 Boston Place, London S.W.1
Ph (01) 262 1128

The British School of Osteopathy
Littlejohn House
1-4 Suffolk Street, London S.W.1
Ph (01) 930 9254
This is Britain's largest and oldest training establishment in complementary and alternative medicine as it has been in London for seventy years. Her Royal Highness Princess Anne is the Patron of the B.S.O.

The British College of Naturopathy and Osteopathy
Fraser House
6 Netherhall Gardens, London
Ph (01) 435 7830

The European School of Osteopathy
104 Tonbridge Road, Maidstone, Kent
Ph (0622) 671 558

The College of Osteopathy
110 Thorkhill Road, Thames Ditton, Surrey
Ph (01) 398 3308

UNITED STATES OF AMERICA
The American Osteopathic Association
142 East Ontario Street, Chicago, Illinois
Ph (312) 280 5800
Osteopathic physicians have full practice rights in all states of America. There are fifteen colleges of osteopathic medicine.

The Hawaiian Osteopathic Association
Dr Alan R. Becker, D.O.
122 Oneawa Street, Kailua Hawaii
Ph (808) 261 6105

CANADA
The Canadian Osteopathic Association
575 Waterloo Street, London,
Ontario
Ph (519) 439 5521

AUSTRALIA
New South Wales
The United Osteopathic Physicians Guild
P.O. Box 620,
Double Bay, Sydney, 2028
Ph (02) 389 3055

The International Colleges of Osteopathy
148 Barker Street,
Randwick, Sydney, 2031
Ph (02) 398 2222
This college incorporates the New South Wales College of Osteopathy
and the Windsor College of Applied Osteopathy. It is accredited by
the U.O.P.G. and the New South Wales Higher Education Board. It
offers a five-year D.O. course in conjunction with the B.Sc. Anatomy
course at the University of New South Wales, adjacent to the college.

The Australian Academy of Osteopathy
Seventh Floor, Beanbah Chambers,
235 Macquarie Street, Sydney 2000
Ph (02) 233 1655

Victoria
The Department of Osteopathic Sciences
Phillips Institute of Technology,
Plenty Road, Bundoora,
Victoria 3083
Ph (03) 468 2596
Clinic (03) 468 2570

The Phillips Institute of Technology offers a five-year degree course of
B.App.Sc. in osteopathy that is accredited by the Australian Osteo-
pathic Association and the General Council and Register of
Osteopaths (U.K.). The osteopathic degree course is recognised by the
Victorian Higher Education Board and funded by the Australian
Government. Students are eligible for tertiary education assistance
grants and full osteopathic registration.

The Australian Osteopathic Association
Kevin Sturges, D.O.
252 Pakington Street,
Geelong, Victoria
Ph (052) 9 8021
This association maintains a register of practitioners mainly in
Victoria and Tasmania.

Queensland
Milton Conn, D.O.
218 Edward Street, Brisbane
Ph (07) 221 8710

John Evans, D.O.
2 Joden Place, Southport
Ph (075) 32 6393

Cameron McGown, D.O.
Sungola Arcade,
153 Scarborough Street, Southport
Ph (075) 32 3013

Patrick Rozanski, B.Sc., D.O.
P.O. Box 600, Mackay
Ph (079) 57 2856 or (079) 57 4065

Keith Trimby, D.O.
227 Sheridan Street, Cairns
Ph (070) 51 4749

South Australia
Douglas Nunn, D.O., Ella Nunn, D.O., and Leslie Nunn, D.O.
15 Franklin Street, Adelaide
Ph (08) 51 4431

Northern Territory
T. Day, D.O.
Tiwi Medical Centre, Rocklands Drive
Tiwi, Darwin
Ph (089) 27 0787

Western Australia
K. Clifford, D.O.
321 Cape Street, Yokine
Ph (09) 349 3679

Andre Gajek, D.O.
Unit 7, 6 Leigh Street,
Victoria Park
Ph (09) 362 3887

Ken R. Grogan, D.O.
Unit 11, 24 Thorogood Street,
Victoria Park
Ph (09) 470 1412

Rosemary A. Latto, D.O.
1 Second Avenue, Mount Claremount
Ph (09) 383 3246

J. Leebold, D.O.
Unit 10, 12 Queen Street,
Perth
Ph (09) 382 4283

H. Moore, M.L.C.O.M.
4 Ventor Avenue, West Perth
Ph (09) 22 5864

NEW ZEALAND
Auckland
The New Zealand Register of Osteopaths Inc.
92 Hurstmere Road,
Takapuna 9
Ph (09) 494 633
A directory of members can be obtained from
P.O. Box 33-768,
Takapuna, Auckland

Coromandel
Will Miller, Ph.D., D.O.
c/o Pauanui P.O.,
Pauanui via Thames

Gerald Whineray, D.O.
200 Karaka Street, Thames
Ph (0843) 89 154

Gisborne
Douglas Sayer, D.O.
Cnr Grafton/Gladstone Road
Ph (079) 85 643

Hastings
Michael Reese, D.O.
707 Frederick Street
Ph (070) 677 55

Napier
Julian Jones, D.O.
42 Munro Street
Ph (070) 588 30

Palmerston North
Richard Robertson, D.O.
86 Victoria Avenue
Ph (063) 772 48

Kevin Barnes, D.O.
72 Rongopai Street
Ph (063) 694 54

Rotorua
William Beetz, D.O.
41 Eruera Street
Ph (073) 827 34

Mark Franken, D.O.
6th Floor B.S.B. Building,
Hinemoa Street
Ph (073) 892 13

South Island
Stephen Joly, D.O.
Worcester Chambers,
69 Worcester Street, Christchurch
Ph (03) 611 31

Chris Rowse, D.O.
As above

Larry Ross, D.O.
94 Riccarton Road, Riccarton
Christchurch
Ph (03) 480 458

Richard Carruthers, D.O.
52 Queens Street,
Blenheim
Ph (057) 831 22

Michael Monaghan, D.O.
Physical Medicine Centre,
5 Examiner Road, Nelson
Ph (054) 84 685

Tauranga
Andrew Wilson, D.O.
59 Seventh Avenue
Ph (075) 834 46

Hella Wilson, D.O.
As above

Te Puke
Jon Henderson, D.O.
1st Floor Professional Chambers,
Jellicoe Street
Ph (075) 360 48

Wayne Tennant-Brown
22 Oxford Street

Waikato
Ron Cook, D.O.
142 Williams Street, Cambridge
Ph (071) 27 8997

Rosemary Cook, D.O.
As above

Whakatane
Noel Williamson, D.O.
45 James Street
Ph (076) 85 285

Whangaparaoa
Anthony Norrie, D.O.
8b Tamariki Avenue, Orewa
Ph (0942) 63 689

Whangarei
Max Belcher, D.O.
2 Grey Street
Ph (089) 483 144

Wellington
Jan Duncan, D.O.
158a Oban Street, Wadestown
Ph (04) 729 766

Judith Thomas, D.O.
As above

Qualifications in Osteopathy

When seeking osteopathic treatment in British Commonwealth countries it is very important to make sure that your practitioner is properly qualified. Although osteopaths are registered, this does not stop unqualified osteopaths and charlatans. Make sure your osteopathic physician has initials appearing after his name that indicate his qualifications and that he is registered.

D.O. – Diploma of Osteopathy or Doctor of Osteopathy
M.N.Z.R.O. – Member of the N.Z. Register of Osteopaths Inc
M.A.O.A. – Member of the Australian Osteopathic Association
M.U.O.P.G. – Member of the United Osteopathic Physicians Guild
M.R.O. – Member of the Register of Osteopaths (U.K.)
M.L.C.O.M. – Member of the London College of Osteopathic Medicine
M.B.N.O.A. – Member of the British Naturopathic and Osteopathic Association
F.A.A.O. – Fellow of the American Academy of Osteopathy.

Due to the legal and social role of osteopathic physicians in the United States, many of them practise only as medical doctors or specialists. Members of the American Academy of Osteopathy are specialists in osteopathic manipulative therapy and foster and develop the distinctive practices of medicine first announced by Dr Still.

BIBLIOGRAPHY

CHAITOW, Leon, *Neuro-Muscular Technique*, Thorsons, 1980

CHAITOW, Leon, *Osteopathy*, Thorsons, 1982

CHAPMAN, Frank, *An Endocrine Interpretation of Chapman's Reflexes*, American Academy of Osteopathy, 1927

HILDRETH, Arthur, *The Lengthening Shadow of Dr Andrew Taylor Still*, Journal Printing Company, 1938

HOAG, J.M., COLE, W.V. and BRADFORD, S.G., *Osteopathic Medicine*, McGraw Hill, 1969

SANDLER, Stephen, *Osteopathy*, Optima, 1987

STILL, Andrew Taylor, *Autobiography*, Journal Printing, 1908

STILL, Andrew Taylor, *Research and Practice*, Journal Printing, 1910

STODDARD, Alan, *The Back — Relief from Pain*, Methuen, 1981

STODDARD, Alan, *A Manual of Osteopathic Technique*, Methuen, 1959

STODDARD, Alan, *A Manual of Osteopathic Practice*, Methuen, 1969

TURNER, Roger Newman, *Naturopathic Medicine*, Thorsons, 1984

UPLEDGER, John, *Osteopathic Doctor's Treasury of Health Secrets*, Parker Publishing, 1974